The Methuselah Factor

Publisher:

COMPASSHEALTH CONSULTING, INC.

FORESTHILL, CALIFORNIA

www.compasshealth.net

Copyright © 2019 by CompassHealth Consulting, Inc.

Published in the United States of America

All Rights Reserved

Edited by Clifford Goldstein

Copy Edited by Gwen Simmons and Sonja DeRose

Graphics by Dhairya Giri

Cover by Julie Burks

Publisher's Notice

ISBN: 978-1-942730-08-8

The Methuselah Factor

Learn How to Live Sharper, Leaner, Longer and Better
—In Thirty Days or Less

By David J. DeRose, MD, MPH

DEDICATION

To the late Bernell Baldwin, PhD, who first introduced me to the wonders of hemorheology.

ABOUT THE AUTHOR

David J. DeRose, MD, MPH

Dr. David DeRose has interspersed public health work for populations and communities with some twenty-five years of clinical practice in Internal Medicine. His nationally syndicated radio show has been airing for some 16 years; it is currently heard on more than 170 stations. DeRose brings solid credentials as a board-certified specialist in both Internal Medicine and Preventive Medicine, in addition to holding a Master of Public Health degree, with an emphasis in Health Promotion and Health Education.

Dr. DeRose's commitment to educating the masses on optimal health strategies has taken him far beyond the radio booth and medical clinic. He has taught at the college level, held numerous seminars for health professionals and lay audiences around the world, and has been featured in TV and video health series. DeRose's research has been published in peer-reviewed medical journals, including *The Journal of the American Medical Association*, *The Annals of Epidemiology*, and *Preventive Medicine*.

FOREWORD

Longevity. Ageless beauty. Immortality. These words identify one of humanity's greatest aspirations. Ponce de Leon's alleged quest for the Fountain of Youth, Alexander the Great's legendary search for a river to remedy senescence, and cross-cultural spiritual aspirations for eternal life—all testify to this enduring human pursuit. Turn back the clock on aging. Live longer and better.

In my three decades as a physician, I've seen these aspirations played out in the lives of my patients, students, and public audiences throughout the world. Indeed, the quest for longevity and high-quality living knows no cultural or geographic boundaries.

Well, with such a pervasive vision, how are we doing?

We have made strides in extending the productive life span. As the numbers of octogenarians and nonagenarians swell, it's obvious we've done at least a few things right. On the other hand, the epidemic of dementia and the surging rates of other chronic conditions like diabetes and obesity remind us that we're still missing many pieces in the optimal longevity puzzle.

Over the years, my work as a board-certified physician in both

Internal Medicine and Preventive Medicine has provided a unique vantage point for surveying practical aspects of the longevity question. Most remarkable has been my clinical experience with intensive lifestyle change programs.

Working with patients in residential health enhancement programs like those offered at Northern California's Weimar Institute[1] and Georgia's Wildwood Lifestyle Center,[2] I've seen remarkable evidence that disease and aging processes can, in many cases, be rapidly reversed. Within two or three weeks, patients with heart disease can often successfully eliminate angina, regain long-lost vigor, and slash their medication bills. In similar short order, individuals with type 2 diabetes or hypertension typically improve blood sugar and blood pressure readings, enhance their well-being, and turn back the clock on their complications—while they too decrease their reliance on prescription drugs. Individuals in the throes of autoimmune diseases like lupus or rheumatoid arthritis can, without adding new medications, sometimes rapidly halt—even reverse—the progression of their conditions. And that's just a sampling of many of the astounding stories that have taken place on the campuses of two institutions that have stood the test of time. (Weimar's NEWSTART program has been operating for more than thirty-five years, and Wildwood has been offering lifestyle-based healing approaches for seventy-five years.)

Although lifestyle approaches are not panaceas, the range of diseases I've seen respond to simple non-drug approaches has convinced me that we've largely overlooked one of the most powerful keys for turning back the clock on disease, poor quality of life, and aging in general. In medical parlance, that key is called "optimizing hemorheology." In lay terms, we're talking about enhancing your blood fluidity—a unifying medical concept that responds very quickly to simple lifestyle strategies.

When I speak before lay audiences, I refer to hemorheology as the "H Factor," or the "Methuselah Factor." The latter designation is inspired by a character in Middle Eastern literature who reputedly was the longest-lived human. I'm convinced that, whatever else he had going for him, Methuselah had great hemorheology.

This book is designed as a practical, how-to guide. In thirty days or less, you'll not only understand many of the important nuances of hemorheology but also skillfully harness this oft-neglected key to longevity and high-quality living. Granted, it's not the Fountain of Youth, but medical science concurs with my clinical experience when I say you're about to embark on a thirty-day journey calculated to help you live longer and better.

CONTENTS

Part One

LAYING THE METHUSELAH FACTOR FOUNDATION

1

A BRIEF OVERVIEW OF HEMORHEOLOGY, THE METHUSELAH FACTOR

LIKE ME, YOU'RE PROBABLY a bit skeptical when you hear about the latest "medical breakthrough." Your skepticism probably increases when you find the touted breakthrough is the subject of another health book or product.

Such skepticism is warranted. Every year volumes of drivel cross my desk, purporting to be the latest panacea or medical breakthrough. There's almost always a significant price tag, even if the purveyors are touting a "natural" product. So, although I'm not selling anything to boost hemorheology (you'll see throughout the pages of this book my practical strategies are extremely cost-effective and require no proprietary agents), I am the author of this volume—and thus, ostensibly, could have something to gain by championing the latest "snake oil."

However, even a quick internet search reveals that hemorheology is bona fide science. Numerous medical societies focus on this and related topics. Selected examples include the Asian Union for Microcirculation, the British Microcirculation Society, the European Society for Clinical Hemorheology and Microcirculation, the German Society for Microcirculation and Vascular Biology, the International Society of Biorheology, the International Society of Clinical Hemorheology, the Israeli Society for Microcirculation, the Italian Society of Clinical Hemorheology and Microcirculation, the Japanese Society of Hemorheology, and the Russian Association for "Regional Haemodynamics and Microcirculation."[3] Furthermore, whole medical journals have been devoted to hemorheology and related sciences. These include *Microcirculation*, *Clinical Hemorheology and Microcirculation*, *Biorheology*, and the *Journal of Biorheology*.

Writing about an established, yet underrecognized, science presents challenges. If I make my case for hemorheology's importance, but by using only very recent research, there's a danger some will think: *This is just a fad; in a few years it will slip off medical research's radar screen.* On the other hand, if I just cite older, established research, others might think hemorheology is no longer a relevant topic. To help address these concerns, I've included a mix of cutting-edge research and time-honored studies. When laying the foundation for hemorheology's importance (Chapters 1 – 13), I've relied more heavily on older, established research. When focused on thirty days of practical strategies (Chapters 14 – 45), I've emphasized the more recent studies.

Like most of my lay audiences, you probably know next to nothing about hemorheology nor even how to pronounce the term. (It's *hee'-moh-ree-ol'-uh-jee*.) However, there are compelling reasons why you should invest the time to learn about this science, which offers incredible promise for enhancing your wellbeing and increasing your lifespan.

What is Hemorheology?

Why all this medical interest in a topic that sounds relatively esoteric? After all, just what is hemorheology?

Merriam-Webster's on-line dictionary defines hemorheology as "the science of the physical properties of blood flow in the circulatory system"[4] A 1985 copy of *Dorland's Medical Dictionary* provided a bit more scholarly definition and further attests that this science is not merely a fad: "the scientific study of the deformation and flow properties of cellular and plasmatic components of blood in the macroscopic, microscopic, and submicroscopic dimensions, and the rheological properties of vessel structure with which the blood comes in direct contact."

In plain English, hemorheology is simply *the science that describes how effectively blood flows throughout your body, nourishing your tissues and eliminating wastes.* In other words, hemorheology is the science of blood fluidity.

Why is Hemorheology Important?

Intuitively, it's probably obvious why we should be interested in optimizing our blood fluidity. Over a century ago—before the nuances of blood flow were understood—a prolific lay health writer captured it this way: "Perfect health depends upon perfect circulation."[5]

This remains a stunningly accurate description of the importance of optimal hemorheology. Modern medical literature is replete with examples of why we should both understand this subject and, then, do our utmost to improve our own blood fluidity. Figure 1 provides a partial listing of some of the more notable benefits of improved hemorheology.

FIGURE 1 Hemorheology, Health, and High-Quality Living

Medical research demonstrates that optimal hemorheology can help address and/or prevent your risk of:

– Stroke

– Coronary Artery Disease

– Blindness (Glaucoma and Macular Degeneration)

– Cancer

– Cognitive Decline

– Hypertension

– Diabetes and Its Complications

– Weight Gain

– Arthritis

– Age-related Physical Deterioration

– Suboptimal Physical Performance Among the Otherwise Young and Fit

If you're ready to improve your Methuselah Factor, great. Whatever questions you might still have, your motivation to embrace *The Methuselah Factor Diet and Lifestyle Program*—and stick with it—will largely reflect your perception of just how important hemorheology is. With that in mind, wherever you're at in the process of getting serious about blood fluidity, the same task beckons.

However, before we take a practical look at the science behind blood fluidity, you'll be best served by something else: an overview of how easy it is to make *The Methuselah Factor Diet and Lifestyle Program* really work for you.

MAKING *THE METHUSELAH FACTOR DIET AND LIFESTYLE PROGRAM* WORK FOR YOU

BEFORE JUMPING INTO THE medical research with both feet, I will explain how *The Methuselah Factor Diet and Lifestyle Program* actually works. First of all, it really is a *program*. I'll give you daily assignments over the course of thirty days that are designed to optimize your blood fluidity. However, the program is *flexible*. Unlike many self-help book authors, I won't lay down a set of rigid prescriptions that you must precisely follow.

From the start, many of you will welcome such a flexible and user-friendly program. However, there's a chance a few of you may look at my program's malleability as a negative. You wanted this doctor-educator to take you by the hand and walk you through a very specific regimen. But that's not, necessarily, in your best interests.

Let me explain. You'll be learning about many ways to improve your blood fluidity—so many, in fact, that I can't pass off a "one size fits all" approach. Granted, some of you are dealing with serious—and, perhaps, life-threatening—medical issues. You'll want to be very serious about each of my recommendations, and will want to incorporate them as quickly as possible, too. For example, you may be looking bariatric surgery square in the face, or dealing with serious diabetic complications, or facing possible heart surgery for coronary artery disease, or struggling with a serious autoimmune condition, or realizing your mental faculties are precipitously slipping.

On the other hand, some of you are not facing any grave medical or physical health issues. Perhaps your energy level has been flagging of late, you're concerned about a family history of cancer, your memory isn't quite as sharp as it used to be, or you're simply trying to hedge your bets that you don't end up like Uncle Ralph with diabetes, high blood pressure and heart disease. You'll also reap benefits from this program, but you might be able to get by with smaller adjustments to your lifestyle.

So, in Part 2 of this book, I'll give you a day-by-day road map for improving your blood fluidity within one month. However, as I challenge you to make daily changes to improve your hemorheology, you'll get to choose how aggressive you want to be. You'll evaluate which changes fit with your lifestyle—and your personal needs. No doubt, you've already picked up on the bottom line: because the Methuselah Factor is so important, the poorer your current health status, the more determined you should be when it comes to rapidly improving your hemorheology.

Program Nuts and Bolts

The core of this book is the day-by-day approach to improving your Methuselah Factor. For each of the thirty days of the program, I'll give you specific insights into hemorheology, and then ask you to apply those principles in your life. Your assignment is to *continue each practice for the entirety of the thirty days.*

In order to fully work the program, you must each day add (or recommit to) a specific diet or lifestyle principle. Yes, that's right, *recommit.* Some of you will find certain tasks easy because they are already a part of your lifestyle. In that situation, all I'm asking is that you recommit to that healthy behavior—and continue to practice it throughout the entire thirty days of the program.

You're in the driver's seat, deciding how much ground to cover during each day of our thirty-day journey. However, make sure to cover some ground each day. That means daily choosing—or recommitting to—the featured lifestyle practice.

Also, although each decision is a commitment for the duration of the thirty days, some of those choices will obligate you to something intermittent in nature. For example, on **Day 7**, I'll ask you to commit to taking a break from your normal routine and focus on recreational activities for just one day per week. Therefore, you'll have to practice that commitment only four times during the thirty-day program. On the other hand, on **Day 12**, you'll make a commitment to drinking a minimum amount of water daily. If you set a goal of eight glasses per day, I'll ask you to drink a minimum of eight glasses of water every day for the rest of the program.

Choosing a Program Start Date

In the next 24 hours you have to choose when you want to start your thirty-day journey toward optimal hemorheology. Ideally, you'll give yourself at least a week to digest the scientific material in the next eleven chapters, Chapters 3 – 13. Those insights really lay the foundation for the program, helping you see just how important the Methuselah Factor is. In fact, if you ever feel your motivation waning, you may want to re-read that material.

However, if you want to start your thirty-day journey sooner, then start by getting at least a quick overview of Chapters 3 – 13, then proceed directly to Chapter 14, where the program essentially begins. Even though you could embark on the journey today, don't neglect at least an attempt, at some point, to seriously read the foundational scientific material. You can read it in installments if you prefer, but you owe it to yourself to understand why hemorheology is so important.

A Few More Words About the Chapters Ahead

The next eleven chapters will be among the most valuable portions of this book for some of you. Perhaps you're a health professional, or a lay person who just loves scientific details. However, for others, there's a chance that some of the scientific minutiae, no matter how well I attempt to explain them, will make your brain spin. Terms like *fibrinogen, von Willebrand factor* and *erythrocyte aggregation* may evoke some of the worst memories from your scholastic years. So, for those of you who don't normally connect with scientific material, I've got good news:

First, in my years teaching college classes, adult education intensives, and other seminars I've gained a reputation for making complex subjects easily understood. In this setting, just like the college classroom, my job is to make this material understandable and have it actually stick. "Dumbing the material down" and talking merely about "thinning your blood" simply won't work. I've been guilty, along with several generations of doctors, of trying to take that easy way out during busy clinic visits. However, the subject of blood fluidity is far more complex than a single sound bite can communicate, which is why the better that you understand what is happening in your body, the easier you'll find it to harness my simple strategies for improving your Methuselah Factor.

Second, if you can't get into all the science stuff, then just skim the next eleven chapters. No tests, no quizzes. However, and this is important—before you start the thirty-day program, you have to be convinced that hemorheology, the Methuselah Factor, is of vital importance. So important, in fact, that you are committed to stick around for the entire month-long journey.

Finally, if you'd like some ancillary video material, my *Longevity Plus* video mini-series gives a good overview of what follows—in addition to beginning to tackle some of the lifestyle strategies that you find beginning in Chapter Fourteen. You can pick up the approximately two-hour series on my website: www. compasshealth.net/purchase.

One Shortcut Not to Take

One other caution is warranted. Don't expect to substitute a simple internet search for the next eleven chapters. There are two reasons for this. First, even a "simple search" using the terms "hemorheology and disease" will likely turn up over 100,000 entries. But second, much of the medical literature that deals with hemorheology never even uses the term (you'll understand why as you continue reading). Therefore, even if you could review all of the medical research that uses the term "hemorheology" you would still be missing the bulk of the scientific evidence.

So let's delve into the science of hemorheology. You'll see what specific factors affect blood fluidity. You'll learn about important connections to optimal health and disease. And most important, you'll begin to understand the power of *The Methuselah Factor Diet and Lifestyle Program*—and obtain a solid foundation for putting it to work in your own life.

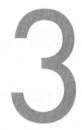

IMPROVE YOUR METHUSELAH FACTOR, DECREASE YOUR RISK OF A STROKE

OVER A DECADE AGO, Hungarian scientists led by Dr. Laszlo Szapary sought to uncover associations between stroke and factors affecting blood fluidity.[6] Their study of nearly 300 patients yielded striking findings. Four key hemorheology-impairing blood factors were connected with stroke (see Figure 2)[7]. Understanding just what those blood factors are will help you not only better appreciate their linkage with stroke, but will also begin to lay the foundation for connecting hemorheology with other disease states.

The type of strokes studied by Szapary and colleagues were of the *ischemic* variety. This designation refers to strokes caused by lack of blood supply to the brain. Such catastrophic events occur when blood vessels to the brain become blocked either by progressive narrowing or by sudden obstruction. An example of the latter scenario occurs when some atherosclerotic debris (think "small piece of a clot"), perhaps from a neck artery (like the carotid), breaks loose and travels to the brain. (Remember all arteries carry blood away from the heart, so blood is flowing in your arteries from your heart *up* to your head).

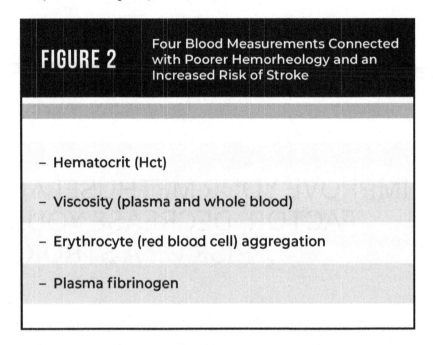

FIGURE 2 — Four Blood Measurements Connected with Poorer Hemorheology and an Increased Risk of Stroke

– Hematocrit (Hct)

– Viscosity (plasma and whole blood)

– Erythrocyte (red blood cell) aggregation

– Plasma fibrinogen

In stark contrast to ischemic strokes are hemorrhagic strokes. These strokes, not studied by Dr. Szapary, result from bleeding into the brain. They can occur when blood vessels rupture from high blood pressure or trauma.

Why did those four implicated blood factors increase the risk of stroke due to blood vessel blockage?

Hematocrit and Stroke

Hematocrit (Hct) refers to the proportion of your blood made up of red blood cells. Having more red blood cells (RBCs) may sound good. This is especially likely if you have a history of anemia, a condition characterized by RBCs that are too few in number and/ or too small in size.

However, a higher hematocrit, more red blood cells in a given volume, can also present problems. Consider the following analogy.

Just as you need red blood cells to carry oxygen to your tissues, so communities need essential public service vehicles to keep their town running smoothly: fire trucks, ambulances, police cars, utility vehicles, garbage trucks, etc. You've got the picture.

So then is a community with more public service vehicles better off? Perhaps, to a point. What happens if you have so many garbage trucks, utility vehicles and police cars clogging your streets that when it comes time to put out a fire, the firefighters can't get there expeditiously?

Although we're talking about a single "vehicle" only, the red blood cell, the illustration still fits. Your arteries and veins—the "roads" of your body—can be clogged by too many RBCs. This is the problem with a high Hct. If too large a percentage of your blood is made up of red blood cells, the red cells do not circulate freely; they get backed up and bottled up. Circulation suffers. And as Dr. Szapary observed, you face a higher risk of stroke.

A powerful illustration of the dangers of high hematocrits comes from the world of elite cycling. Regardless of your interest in professional bicycling, most of us have heard reports describing the history of "blood doping" in this sport.[8] The evidence indicates that one of the favored practices involved artificially increasing Hct. Before the advent of today's powerful medications, this was sometimes accomplished through autologous transfusions (literally blood transfusions that you give to yourself).

How?

Let's say you're a professional cyclist competing in the 1980s. You've heard that having a higher Hct can help you carry more oxygen in your blood. (This appears to be true, incidentally.[9]) So, two months before the big race, you see your friendly accomplice, a physician. Doc proceeds to withdraw a pint of your blood. He adds the appropriate preservatives to your recent donation, and puts it into a special refrigerator.

A month later you're back in the same clinic. Over the past thirty days, you've built up your Hct, close to where it was some four weeks earlier. Now Doc steps into the picture again. You part with another pint of blood. It ends up in that same refrigerator.

Finally, just a few days before the race, you pay a final visit to Doc's office. This time you don't "donate" any blood. You're there for an autologous transfusion. That's right. You're there to be reinfused with two pints of *your own blood*.

On race day, evidence indicates your now substantially higher hematocrit will allow you to carry more oxygen and perform better, but—at a price: your hemorheology has been greatly compromised. With a greatly heightened risk of stroke (and heart attack as we'll see in the next section), you engage in the competition.

Although many blood dopers seemed to fare fairly well, others paid the ultimate price. A number of elite cyclist deaths have been attributed to autologous transfusions—or to Hct-raising treatment with a younger cousin, EPO injections.[10] (EPO or erythropoietin is a hormone that causes your bone marrow to make more blood cells, thus raising your hematocrit without all the mess of autologous transfusions.)

Yes, higher hematocrits have some advantages, but when it comes to circulatory disorders, too high can be downright dangerous. We'll look at just how high is too high later in this book. However, there's a final chapter in the stroke-hematocrit story that first begs to be told.

A little over a year after Dr. Szapary and associates made the connection between high Hct and an increased risk of stroke, a team of Australian researchers upped the ante as far as the risks of living with a high hematocrit. Lead author Dr. Louise Allport reported that higher Hcts carried another danger in the setting of a stroke: more devastating and less reversible brain damage.[11]

Reviewing Szapary's other hemorheology-stroke connections (those involving viscosity, RBC aggregation, and fibrinogen) amounts to far more than a mere academic exercise. These very same players will surface repeatedly as we seek to optimize our Methuselah Factor. So, let's take a few more minutes to get acquainted with some of the other actors in the hemorheology drama.

Viscosity and Stroke

As would any good physician, I practice what I preach. So, right now I'm interspersing my writing with draughts from my water bottle. (If you haven't already guessed, we'll learn that keeping well hydrated is one important way to optimize your Methuselah Factor.)

If you were sitting in my office and observed me downing a good quantity of water, I would turn to you and pose the following question: "Did that fluid I just imbibed look like it had high or low viscosity?" If you understand the concept of viscosity, "the property of a fluid or semi-fluid that resists flow," then you would have correctly identified my favorite beverage as having low viscosity. If I then tried the same demonstration with olive oil, maple syrup, and finally molasses, you would witness me swallowing progressively more viscous fluids (and likely getting sick in the process).

In medical circles we sometimes measure the viscosity of something called *plasma*. Plasma is simply the liquid portion of blood (i.e., blood with the red blood cells, white blood cells and platelets removed). Alternately, we can measure whole blood viscosity, which includes those various cellular elements.

In Szapary's research, both plasma and whole blood viscosity were linked to greater risk of cerebrovascular diseases like strokes. This should now be fairly intuitive. Anything that causes your blood to flow less freely, like greater viscosity, could impair optimal blood flow to vital regions such as your brain.

Erythrocyte Aggregation and Stroke

Erythrocyte is a fancy name for a red blood cell (abbreviated RBC). Szapary and colleagues found something else that shouldn't be surprising. Namely, if one's red blood cells tend to clump together, he or she will experience an increased risk of stroke.

This also shouldn't be difficult to conceptualize if you understand a key relationship between your red blood cells and your blood vessels. Namely, the diameter of your RBCs (approximately 8 microns) is larger than the diameter of your smallest blood vessels (you have capillaries as small as 3 microns[12]).

Let me illustrate. Some years ago, I was driving a sedan through an alley in Europe. I noticed that the alley was getting progressively smaller until I reached a point where it was obvious that soon the width of that shrinking thoroughfare would be smaller than the width of my car. Needless to say, I promptly backed out. However, what would have happened had a dozen cars been following me?

This gives you a glimpse of what is happening in your circulatory system every instant. RBCs come to "alleys" that are smaller in diameter than they are. However, those red cells cannot back up. Literally millions of RBCs are lined up behind them—and all flow is unidirectional, thanks to your ever-functioning heart. What, then, spares us from circulatory gridlock in our tiny vessels?

The amazing answer is this: your red blood cells are more malleable than was that European sedan I rented. In my case, driving further would only have ensured that a metal vehicle got pinned between two opposing walls. When it comes to your RBCs, they can fold on themselves and *squeeze through* tiny capillaries.

This remarkable feat is accomplished, in part, through the design of your red cells. Their unique shape is technically called a biconcave disc (see Figure 3). In plain English, your RBCs are shaped like donuts—with one major difference. Instead of having a hole in the middle they have a thinner central region. This novel shape allows for impressive folding and squeezing.

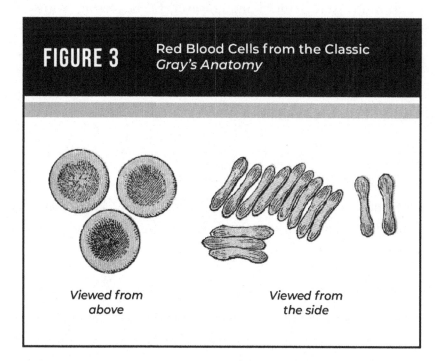

FIGURE 3 Red Blood Cells from the Classic *Gray's Anatomy*

Viewed from above

Viewed from the side

However, a couple of things can bring your red cells' acrobatics to an abrupt halt. One of them is stiff membranes. Two decades before Szapary's work, evidence was accumulating that more rigid red cell membranes were associated with greater risk of stroke.[13] More recent research has connected stiffer RBCs in the early morning hours with an increased risk of heart attack and stroke.[14]

The other show stopper is erythrocyte aggregation. If your red cells clump together, their malleability will be of little avail. Those clumps of red cells will not be able to optimally negotiate your blood vessels—and, as the Hungarian researchers found, that circulatory compromise will increase your risk of stroke.

In other words, the Szapary research tells us at least three things. If you want to avoid strokes, keep your hematocrit at a reasonable level, decrease your viscosity, and keep your red blood cells from becoming too sticky. Granted, this is not a particularly useful prescription—yet. Before long, however, I'll be sharing with you the simple lifestyle steps that can help you effect these changes.

But before we do that, we've still got to add the final piece to the stroke puzzle.

Plasma Fibrinogen and Stroke

Most lay people have heard of red blood cells. The concept of viscosity is widely used outside of medicine. Even if you didn't know exactly what hematocrit was before reading this chapter, there's a good chance the term actually sounded familiar. However, most of my lay audiences have never heard of the final factor that the Szapary team linked to stroke: fibrinogen.

Fibrinogen is a clotting protein. If you've never studied how blood clots, I'll spare you the detailed medical school version. However, it is an amazingly orchestrated process. One of the key players in the clotting symphony is fibrinogen. Also known as clotting factor I, fibrinogen is activated when you need to stop bleeding; for example, after accidentally cutting your finger. In such a scenario, your body converts fibrinogen into a related protein called fibrin, which forms the basis for a clot.

With this in mind, it's not difficult to imagine that fibrin would impair blood flow. However, why would a not-yet-activated protein like fibrinogen undermine optimal hemorheology? The reasons are complex. However, fibrinogen exerts its effects, at least in part, by influencing two components we have already studied: red blood cell aggregation and viscosity.

A few years ago, Korean researchers nicely summarized the relationship between fibrinogen and red cell clumping. They explained how, in the smaller blood vessels, "Fibrinogen molecules form a cross-linking network structure, encouraging erythrocyte [RBC] aggregation."[15] Apparently, due at least in part to this cross-linking, RBCs tend to clump together while blood viscosity also increases.

So, there you have it. Four key hemorheology factors are linked to stroke. Right now, that may seem like more than you ever wanted to know. However, we've not only made some important connections with longevity and high-quality living, we've also laid some important groundwork. We're now ready to tackle much more efficiently ten other vital linkages with the Methuselah Factor, hemorheology.

4

IMPROVE YOUR METHUSELAH FACTOR, DECREASE YOUR RISK OF A HEART ATTACK

CONNECTIONS BETWEEN HEMORHEOLOGY AND coronary artery disease, the cause of heart attacks, have long been reported in the medical literature. It takes no great leap of logic to realize that the same factors that increase our risk of blockage in our brain arteries (the cause of ischemic stroke) would also increase our risk of heart artery blockages (the cause of heart attacks).

For over three decades, researchers in the U.K. have been gathering data on heart disease risk factors from a representative sample of men from Caerphilly in South Wales and Speedwell (a district of Bristol, England). The researchers found that, in as little as five years, hemorheologic factors influenced life and death outcomes.[16] Figure 4 reveals a strong connection between heart attacks and two of our new friends (fibrinogen and plasma viscosity). Note that these compounds conferred huge increases in risk. Those with the highest levels of fibrinogen or viscosity had approximately four times the likelihood of a major heart event when compared to those with the lowest levels.

In that same figure you will note one new player, white blood cell count, showed a similar, but slightly less marked connection. (Still, being in the highest fifth of the population for white count tripled one's risk of a heart event.)

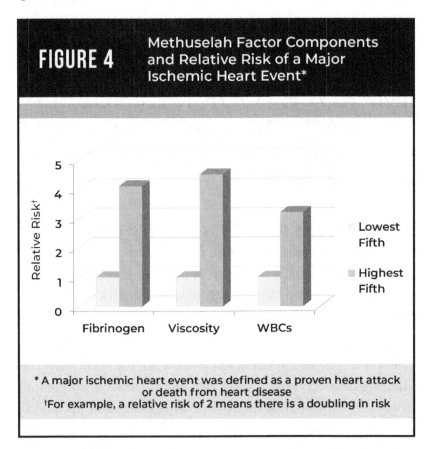

FIGURE 4 Methuselah Factor Components and Relative Risk of a Major Ischemic Heart Event*

* A major ischemic heart event was defined as a proven heart attack or death from heart disease
†For example, a relative risk of 2 means there is a doubling in risk

At this point, I don't expect any surprises on the fibrinogen or viscosity fronts—but what about white blood cells (WBCs)? Aren't these the good guys that are supposed to help us fight infection?

It's true: we need WBCs to ward off bacterial invaders. However, higher WBC counts (you may have guessed) also worsen hemorheology. The evidence suggests that if you want optimal circulatory health, you should opt for a low normal white count rather than a higher level. (Incidentally, the *Methuselah Factor Diet and Lifestyle* is virtually guaranteed to lower your WBC count significantly—which you now realize is a good thing, not a cause for concern.)

Over a decade after the aforementioned publication, Dr. Yarnell and his colleagues came out with an even more stunning conclusion. Now with over 10 years of data under their belts, they announced to the medical community that by measuring Methuselah Factor variables like WBCs, fibrinogen, and viscosity, they could predict heart disease risk with equal or greater precision than if they had measured conventional heart risk factors like total cholesterol, HDL, and triglycerides.[17] Five years later, Italian researchers extended their observations. Even if you had a heart attack, the heart attack was likely to be more serious and extensive if your blood fluidity was worse, as indicated by factors like a higher WBC count and poorer blood viscosity.[18] More recent research continues to confirm and strengthen these associations.[19]

Do you see the point? If you are serious about lowering your risk of heart events, you can't be content with merely managing your cholesterol. The data emphatically states you must be concerned about your blood fluidity.

If that data isn't compelling enough, here's more.

Most emergency room doctors know that heart attacks (technically, myocardial infarctions or MIs) don't occur with equal frequency throughout the day. Although things like mental stress or physical exertion can trigger an event, other things being equal, you're much more likely to have an MI in the morning than after noon. Figure 5 contains data from over 66,000 heart attack patients.[20]

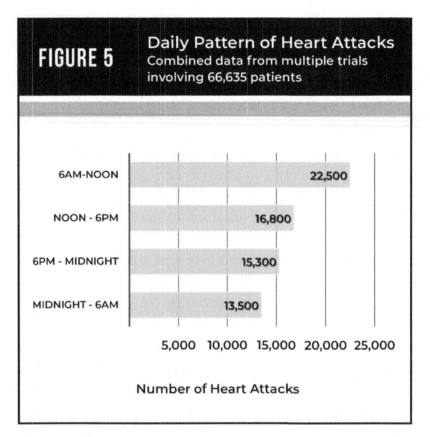

FIGURE 5

Daily Pattern of Heart Attacks
Combined data from multiple trials
involving 66,635 patients

6AM-NOON	22,500
NOON - 6PM	16,800
6PM - MIDNIGHT	15,300
MIDNIGHT - 6AM	13,500

5,000 10,000 15,000 20,000 25,000

Number of Heart Attacks

Notice that, when the day was divided into quarters, nearly 6000 more MIs occurred during the hours of 6 AM and noon than any other six-hour block. Expressed another way, approximately 10% of the heart attacks seemed to be related to something unique about the morning hours.

So what does all this have to do with hemorheology? Everything. Research reveals that blood fluidity is at its very worst in the morning (before breakfast). In contrast, optimal values occur around 1:30 PM.[21]

Over two decades ago, European researchers Wolfgang Koenig and Edzard Ernst put it this way: "Evidence from experimental, clinical and epidemiological studies suggest, that several hemostatic and hemorheological factors (e.g., fibrinogen, Factor VII, plasma viscosity, hematocrit, red blood cell aggregation, total white cell count) might not only play an important role in the evolution of acute thrombotic events, but may also take part in the pathophysiology of atherosclerosis."[22] In other words, well over twenty years ago, these experts were suggesting that the very factors we've been looking at were involved not only in triggering things like heart attack and stroke ("acute thrombotic events") but were also involved in what is called the "pathophysiology" or root causes of these atherosclerotic diseases. If speaking to a lay audience they may well have paraphrased their insights, "These Methuselah Factor components seem to be causing the very development of blockages in arteries ('atherosclerosis')."

But Koenig and Ernst weren't finished. They concluded, "Deeper insight into the mechanisms involved might lead to new preventive strategies as well as to therapeutic procedures in the management of atherosclerosis and associated thrombotic events."

Well, that deeper insight has arrived. The resounding message is this: The Methuselah Factor, hemorheology, is of extreme importance when it comes to your heart.

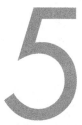

IMPROVE YOUR METHUSELAH FACTOR, DECREASE YOUR RISK OF VISUAL IMPAIRMENT

AFTER LOOKING AT LIFE-THREATENING diseases like heart attack and stroke, blindness may seem a bit mundane. After all, have you ever heard of anyone dying from visual impairment? (If you're thinking Aunt Nellie died from blindness when she walked in front of that car—or off a cliff, forget it. She died from trauma. Her blindness was only a contributory factor.) But such dialogue really misses the point. The Methuselah Factor contributes not only to longevity but also to quality of life. And vision is a big contributor to high-quality living.

The bottom line is this: medical research convincingly links impaired blood fluidity with an increased risk of vision loss. In Chapter 9 we'll probe connections between hemorheology and diabetes—the leading cause of visual impairment among adults in the Western world. If you never develop diabetes, some of the most likely conditions to rob you of vision are glaucoma and macular degeneration. These disorders are also linked to poor blood fluidity.

This topic is a serious matter, even if you're currently unaware of any eye problems. I was reminded of this some years ago in a very unusual setting. While lecturing in Minnesota, I was housed in a guest room on an academic campus. The room was tastefully furnished, but featured some of the most unique décor I had ever witnessed: the room was full of Minnesota Twins baseball memorabilia.

Many players from Twins teams over the years were represented. However, one face recurred with striking frequency. Whether it was an artistic print, a poster, or a team picture, there he was: Kirby Puckett. Although not much of a baseball aficionado, I had heard of Kirby. But when you end up spending more than a week in a room with a guy (or at least facsimiles of him), you want to know a bit more about your roommate.

A quick internet search revealed the reason for Kirby's prominence in that Minnesota venue. I learned among other things that he was "the Twins' all-time leader in career hits, runs, doubles, and total bases" and helped lead them to two World Series victories.[23] However, I also was brought fairly quickly into my own element, the world of medicine. Kirby's playing career was cut short due to complications from glaucoma. As best I could piece the story together, one morning during spring training, that previously undiagnosed condition contributed to something called a "central retinal vein occlusion" and the precipitous loss of vision in one eye. Three surgeries couldn't restore his sight.

Vision in only one eye may seem adequate for most of us, but for a baseball player it is career-ending. Without two functional eyes you lose the majority of your depth perception. Kirby

Puckett's tragic career-ending disorder reminds us that glaucoma, like macular degeneration, can rob us of sight in short order.

So just what are these two conditions, and how are they connected with the Methuselah Factor?

Glaucoma is a condition that damages your optic nerve, "the electrical conduit" that carries visual information from your eye to your brain. Although typically associated with increased pressure in the eye itself, glaucoma can occur with eye pressure readings that are technically normal.

Worldwide research has testified for years that worsened blood fluidity increases your risk of this often insidious sight-robbing condition. For example, over two decades ago, the Canadian research literature reported on a comparison between individuals with glaucoma and those with normal eyes. Those with glaucoma revealed significantly worse blood viscosity.[24] A subsequent Chinese study found that glaucoma was associated not only with worsened blood and plasma viscosity but also with other markers of poorer blood fluidity such as higher levels of hematocrit and fibrinogen, and a greater tendency toward red blood cell aggregation.[25] Other international investigators have made similar observations.[26]

Sound familiar? That's right, the same things that increase a person's risk of a potentially life-threatening or crippling stroke also stack the deck against you when it comes to glaucoma.

However, the blood fluidity-vision saga doesn't end there. Another leading cause of adult blindness, macular degeneration, is also linked to poor hemorheology. Before looking at the research, let's ensure we all understand the nature of this condition.

Some 2 million Americans over 40 years old have age-related macular degeneration (AMD). In this condition, damage occurs to the most sensitive part of one's retina, a region called the macula, which is essential for optimal central vision. (Central vision is involved when you look directly at something. This stands in contrast to peripheral vision which is responsible for the outskirts of your visual field).

Like glaucoma, AMD can gradually erode your visual capacity. And it is no bit player. AMD now heads the list of leading causes of impaired close vision (think *reading and writing*) among those 65 and older.

When it comes to blood fluidity and AMD, the data is again impressive. Consider the findings of British ophthalmologists who compared nearly 80 men and women suffering from age-related macular degeneration with 25 of their visually-healthy peers.[27] Those with AMD had higher levels of a variety of blood fluidity-impairing factors, which included the now-familiar plasma viscosity and fibrinogen. The British investigators also documented increased levels of something called the von Willebrand factor (vWF) among the AMD patients.

Von Willebrand factor is another important clotting factor. Like fibrinogen, white blood cells, and red blood cells, having this blood constituent in sufficient amounts is requisite for circulatory health; too much, however, impairs optimal blood fluidity.

Clearly the evidence from eye health pleads: if you value your vision, be serious about your Methuselah Factor.

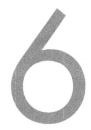

IMPROVE YOUR METHUSELAH FACTOR, DECREASE YOUR RISK OF CANCER

ALL WE'VE EXAMINED TO this point may sound quite logical. In a nutshell we've seen that diseases which result from severe circulatory disturbance, like heart attack and stroke, are related to factors that affect your circulation.

When it comes to sight-impairing conditions like glaucoma and macular degeneration, the connection with hemorheological factors may not seem so intuitive. However, when you realize that eye health is largely dependent on high quality circulation to the back of the eye, called the retina, most lay people are not surprised to learn the Methuselah Factor, hemorheology, has a bearing on vision.

But now the plot really thickens as we turn our attention to cancer. Could factors influencing blood fluidity really influence our risk of malignancy and its ravages?

The year was 2000. The county was Germany. The journal was

Clinical Hemorheology and Microcirculation (one from which I've been quoting liberally, if you hadn't noticed my references). The team, led by Georg-Friedrich von Tempelhoff, was looking for connections between hemorheologic factors and cancer among 451 women undergoing surgery for female malignancies (e.g., ovary, breast, and cervix).[28]

As they followed these women postoperatively, they made some obvious, but other startling, discoveries.

In the obvious category, von Tempelhoff's team found that women with poor blood fluidity, indicated by increased plasma viscosity, were more likely to have "thrombosis" or blood clotting. No surprises there.

However, if you're new to the importance of the Methuselah Factor, the following would clearly come under the "startling" heading. Pre-operative measurement of plasma viscosity was a predictor of long-term survival in women with both ovarian and breast cancer. The researchers also found a connection between red cell aggregation (remember, the tendency of RBCs to clump together) and female cancers.

Why these connections? Listen to the authors' own words— and then I'll paraphrase. "In gynecologic cancer patients the combination of an increase in RBC aggregation and plasma viscosity impairs blood-flow-properties and may induce hypoxia in the microcirculation that favors thrombosis, settlement of tumor-cells and thus metastasis."

What von Tempelhoff's team was saying is simply this: poorer hemorheology (indicated by things like red blood cell aggregation and plasma viscosity) tends to affect oxygen delivery through your smallest blood vessels (i.e., "hypoxia in the microcirculation"). This in turn sets the stage for the formation of tiny clots ("thrombosis"). Tumor cells can then lodge in those clots, relatively isolated from the circulatory system with its immune cells, and gain a foothold for metastasis, the spread of the cancer.

We could look at many other examples that make a similar case for a connection between hemorheology and the spread of cancer, with resultant increased risk of mortality. However, in the cancer research literature, these connections are so compelling that by 2010 another European research team could summarize, "The association between cancer and haemostasis [a similar term referring to the Methuselah Factor or hemorheology], as well as inflammation, is widely accepted."[29] They went on to say unequivocally, "Extensive studies on human and animal tumour biology indicate a specific link between fibrinogen and the progressive and metastatic behaviour of tumour cells." That their comments were limited to fibrinogen was not surprising. The research paper in question was limited to cancer connections with this single Methuselah Factor component. However, I could just as well have chosen other hemorheology factors like viscosity or RBC aggregation that were tracked by von Tempelhoff's team.

By now the point should be clear. Once you've received the diagnosis of cancer, the research literature indicates you should be very concerned about your Methuselah Factor. However, what about those who've never had cancer? Does hemorheology have any connection with what we physicians call "primary cancers"— or cancers that arise for the first time (not spread from somewhere else)?

In 2010, medical researchers from the University of Arkansas made a significant contribution to the literature on the topic of the Methuselah Factor and cancer. Lead author Shashank Jain and colleagues reviewed the scientific literature relating to this topic.[30] They answered our most recent question in the affirmative, finding that Methuselah Factor components increased the risk not only of the spread of cancer but also of developing it in the first place. Some of their findings are summarized in Figure 6.

FIGURE 6	Examples of Hemorheologic Factors Connected with Cancer Risk
Cancer Type	Factor Implicated
Primary	Thrombin
Metastatic	Thrombin, Fibrinogen, Platelet Count

We've already looked at enough data to realize that the case is solid regarding a cancer-Methuselah Factor connection. But the Arkansas team mentioned a couple of other hemorheologic factors worth noting.

Thrombin, as indicated in Figure 6, is linked to both primary and metastatic cancer. Like fibrinogen, it is a protein involved in the clotting process. In fact, it is thrombin that converts fibrinogen into the active clotting compound known as fibrin. Greater amounts of thrombin in your body worsen hemorheology—and increase your risk of cancer. When we look at how *The Methuselah Factor Diet and Lifestyle Program* can improve your blood fluidity, we'll want to keep our eyes open for factors that decrease thrombin as well as other components that worsen our hemorheology. In fact, we'll learn about some amazing linkages between the type and quantity of our fat intake and our thrombin levels.

The other important clotting component spotlighted by Jain and colleagues was the platelet. These "cells" (or, some would say more technically, cell fragments—because they lack nuclei) are vital when it comes to our ability to prevent bleeding. If seriously deficient in platelets, you can bleed to death. For example, a relatively minor surgical procedure could result in a life-threatening bleeding episode. A platelet-deficient person can also begin bleeding spontaneously from places like the nose, mouth or bowels.

On the other hand, having more platelets than optimal is a significant risk factor for cancer and other conditions related to poor hemorheology.

On the malignancy front, these cells have some startling properties. For example, when platelets are found in excess, or if those you have in moderate amounts are more active than they should be, they can literally hide metastatic cancer cells from your body's immune system.

Platelets are tiny, only about 2-3 microns in their greatest diameter. In contrast, cancer cells can have diameters that are tenfold larger—or more.[31] This translates to cancer cell volumes that might be 1000 times greater than those of the tiny platelets. How in the world could such tiny cells hide such giant ones?

Perhaps a simple illustration will suffice. Could you use a leaf to hide a military tank in the forest? You're likely thinking, *Of course not.* However, if you covered that tank with many leaves from many trees, you might hide that tank or even a larger object.

The same is true with platelets. These tiny cells, if found in large enough amounts and activated sufficiently, can actually coat cancer cells so effectively that they are "camouflaged" from your immune system.

Why is this so important? Most cancers release cells into the blood stream, setting the stage for metastasis. However, animal models of how cancer spreads reveal that special white blood cells called Natural Killer (NK) Cells will gobble up 99.99% of the malignant cells before they can lodge anywhere.[32] Even those that escape this line of defense and gain a foothold in a distant organ can be eliminated by a healthy immune system.

Now enter the platelet. An abundance of activated platelets can literally sequester or hide the blood-borne cancer cells from your NK defenders. Result: increased rates of metastasis.

What, then, activates platelets? One of the factors is none other than thrombin itself. As Jain and colleagues put it, "thrombin treatment of platelets facilitates platelet adhesion on tumor cells by 2- to 4-fold in various cancer cells."

Another platelet-activating factor is something called oxidation.[33] Consequently, one of the key elements of *The Methuselah Factor Diet and Lifestyle Program* is antioxidant-rich food items. This will tend to keep your platelets more docile, leading to better hemorheology and a more favorable internal environment when it comes to cancer prevention.

The plot continues to thicken. A host of factors that worsen hemorheology also increase our likelihood of experiencing cancer or dying from the ravages of it. Thrombin, platelet count, and fibrinogen are just some of the bad actors.

7

IMPROVE YOUR METHUSELAH FACTOR, IMPROVE YOUR MENTAL CLARITY AND DECREASE YOUR RISK OF DEMENTIA

IF YOU'RE NOT CONCERNED about your risk of stroke, heart disease, vision loss or cancer, then at least be concerned about cognitive decline. And the research is equally compelling: worsen your blood fluidity, and you'll worsen your brain performance.

A couple of examples should suffice. Both come from the research team studying the Caerphilly cohort of men who, at the time of a 2001 publication, were between the ages of 55 and 69.[34] Dr. Peter Elwood and his British colleagues first made some fascinating observations about hematocrit (Hct) and brain function. (You'll recall that hematocrit is the percentage of your blood made up of red blood cells.)

The investigators looked at how Hct affected something called choice reaction time (CRT). CRT is a very practical measurement. It quantitates how quickly someone can evaluate a cue and then make an appropriate decision. This cognitive skill is utilized in many real-life situations. For example, let's say that you decide to visit me in my Northern California home. Due to travel delays, you end up on the road far later than you hoped. You're driving the last stretch of the road in total darkness.

Then a deer dashes in front of you. At that moment, you have to make a choice: do you hit the brakes or swerve and try to miss the deer? How quickly you act is a measure of cognitive functioning.

So how do they test for this in a lab? It's simple. In one popular version of the test, the subject sits at a computer. He is rapidly shown a series of colored circles on one or the other side of the monitor (see Figure 7).

If the test subject is shown the yellow circle on the left, he is instructed to hit the "Z" key (on the left-hand side of the keyboard) as fast as possible. However, if he is shown a blue circle on the right-hand side of the screen, he must attempt, just as rapidly, to hit the "/" key (on the right side of the keyboard). Thus, a person's score (his response time in milliseconds) is inversely proportional to his cognitive processing. In other words, a higher score (more time taken) would indicate worse performance; in contrast, a lower score reflects better cognitive functioning.

The Caerphilly test was more complicated. Participants had to use a special key pad to indicate into which of four different boxes a star appeared. But you get the idea about how the test works. Most importantly you understand the goal is a lower score, not a higher one. With this background, you can now appreciate the Caerphilly findings as illustrated in Figure 8.

The bottom line is this: too low a hematocrit is bad for cognitive performance, but so is one that's too high. Neither finding

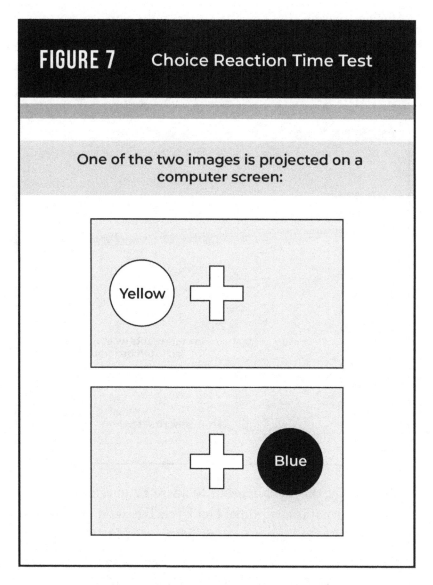

FIGURE 7 Choice Reaction Time Test

One of the two images is projected on a computer screen:

Yellow

Blue

should be surprising. If Hct is too low, you have too few RBCs to carry sufficient oxygen to your brain. In this relatively oxygen-deficient state, performance suffers. On the other extreme, too high an Hct worsens your Methuselah Factor. This, too, undermines oxygen delivery to the brain. This time the problem is not insufficient oxygen carriers, but rather traffic jams in your micro-circulation caused by more RBCs than optimal.

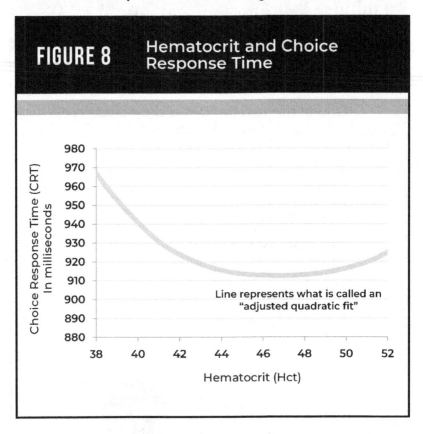

FIGURE 8 Hematocrit and Choice Response Time

By the way, this data helps us to answer a question raised earlier. Namely, what is an optimal Hct level? Based on the Caerphilly cohort, the best readings were somewhere around 46.

Dr. Ellwood's team didn't stop their search for linkages between the Methuselah Factor and mental performance with hematocrit. They also measured plasma viscosity. Based on your expanding acumen regarding things hemorheological, you may already anticipate the results.

In contrast to hematocrit, where optimal scores were in the middle range, "plasma viscosity showed strong and robust relationships, with significantly better cognitive performance and faster reaction times at lower levels of viscosity."[35] No surprises, right? Lower viscosity yields better blood flow and better cognitive performance.

You might be wondering what all this has to do with dementia. After all, I made a tacit promise in the chapter title that I'd be connecting the dots between hemorheology and this condition. To this point in the chapter I've already been providing you with some compelling evidence that such a connection indeed exists. Let me explain why.

Over time, we all experience some deterioration in cognitive processing, whether or not it significantly impacts our lives. Therefore, one key to avoiding dementia (a condition diagnosed when a person has life-impairing deficits in memory and other cognitive functions), is to optimize our cognitive powers. The better our cognitive functioning today, the less any gradual deterioration will noticeably affect our mental performance tomorrow.

But there's far more to the dementia-hemorheology connection. For example, there is a strong connection between Methuselah Factor abnormalities and Alzheimer's disease.[36] However, rather than go into any additional detail here, I'll leave you with a promise. Once we get into our practical, thirty-day program, I'll roll out more insights into dementia prevention, all in the context of practical things that you can do to preserve your mental faculties. Can't wait until then? Then feel free to quickly scan Chapters 24 and 30 for further insights into how paying attention to your Methuselah Factor offers the promise of helping you stave off dementia.

I could say a lot more about brain function and the Methuselah Factor. I could bolster those conclusions with more scientific data. However, by now the point should be clear. What's good for your heart, your eyes, and cancer prevention is also best for brain performance. You want to optimize your blood fluidity for maximal cognitive prowess—now and in the future.

8

IMPROVE YOUR METHUSELAH FACTOR, IMPROVE YOUR BLOOD PRESSURE

HEALTHY AND FLEXIBLE BLOOD vessels are one of the keys to good blood pressure. Conversely, when your small arteries and their lining cells, known as the "endothelium" are in poor shape, those circulatory conduits become stiffer. Additionally, unhealthy lining cells ("endothelial cells") are incapable of making sufficient amounts of nitric oxide gas, a natural blood vessel relaxant. (That's right. Healthy blood vessels actually make a gas that works to relax the very vessels that produce the gas.)

Why are stiffer, less-relaxed blood vessels a problem when it comes to high blood pressure? Consider the following analogy. You are throwing a birthday party for a six-year old and want to do it right. And you decide doing a kid's birthday right means balloons—lots of them.

So you're off to your local party-supply retailer. Once in the store you begin talking with an employee about the 1000 balloons you want. You're determined not to succumb to any of the sales pressure to buy a helium canister or an air compressor to aid you in the task. After all, you've been reading *The Methuselah Factor* and want to showcase your newfound powers. "Thank you, I'll be blowing up all thousand balloons using mere lung power," you reply.

However, you've still got a major decision before you. Do you want the heavier-grade balloons, which are stiffer and less capable of distention? Or do you want the thinner-grade balloons that have less resistance to filling? With the prospect of inflating 1000 balloons, you reason the ones easier to distend should get the nod. You'll have to expend less air pressure per balloon to get the job done.

Well, the same is true with your heart. If your blood vessels are stiff, your heart will have to generate considerably more pressure to fill your arteries with blood. In fact, there's a simple rule of thumb in the medical community: higher resistance to flow in the small vessels, higher blood pressure.

Now, in case you're still cogitating on that balloon analogy, the metaphor eventually breaks down. It's possible you were thinking you would choose the heavier-grade balloons because of their greater resistance to bursting during the inevitable melee that will ensue when forty 6-year-old boys and girls fill your home.

Well, here's a situation where what's good for balloons is not good for blood vessels. It's typically the stiffer, unhealthy blood vessels that are most prone to develop aneurysms (defects that cause them to bulge and potentially rupture) as opposed to normal healthy vessels. In other words, stiff blood vessels or ones that otherwise have difficulty relaxing (e.g., because their lining cells cannot produce sufficient amounts of nitric oxide) are never your friends.

Enter hemorheology. Anything that worsens blood flow in your small blood vessels decreases oxygen delivery to the endothelial cells and puts them under what is called "oxidative stress." When those lining cells are thus stressed, nitric oxide production falls, rendering your tiny arteries less distensible. Your heart will, then, likely compensate by generating higher blood pressures.[37]

This is not mere theory. Researchers for years have been demonstrating connections between a poor Methuselah Factor and high blood pressure. For example, in 1999 Italian researchers, Cicco and Pirrelli, studied 320 patients.[38] They found those with hypertension had several hallmarks of poor blood fluidity, including a greater tendency toward RBC aggregation and higher fibrinogen levels. Of additional import, the researchers measured tissue oxygenation using a transcutaneous oximeter (a device placed on the skin of the areas in question). They found that the hemorheologic abnormalities were associated with poorer tissue oxygenation. And remember: poor oxygenation of the endothelium leads to less distensible arteries and high blood pressure.

In 2012, lead author Hiroko Sugimori and his Japanese colleagues summarized their research into other aspects of the Methuselah Factor literature in these words: "increase in blood viscosity, platelet activation, or both is presumed to play a part in the pathogenesis [cause] of hypertension [high blood pressure]."[39]

If you don't feel you can make it through another five chapters before learning at least *something* to improve your hemorheology, perhaps this is the time to give you a glimpse into one aspect of *The Methuselah Factor Diet and Lifestyle Program*. This is an appropriate juncture because it actually answers a question some of you might be asking.

If you're reading this book, you may have been exposed to an earlier thirty-day program that I helped publicize. Along with physician Greg Steinke and nurse practitioner Trudie Li, I penned a book that still ranks among Amazon's top titles on high blood pressure, *Thirty Days to Natural Blood Pressure Control*. If you read that book, you might be surprised by all this talk about the Methuselah Factor—especially when it comes to high blood pressure. Perhaps you've even gone so far as electronically searching the Kindle edition of *Thirty Days to Natural Blood Pressure Control* and confirmed your suspicions: the word *hemorheology* never appeared in my earlier work. So, did I and my co-authors keep something back from you, all the while pretending we were giving you a comprehensive blood pressure program?

Not at all. We discussed hemorheology but used the more lay-friendly term of *blood fluidity*. One place we explored some of these relationships was in our chapter dealing with beverages. There we highlighted the blood-fluidity-enhancing properties of water. (Yes, if you haven't gathered as much already, drinking plenty of pure water is one of the pillars of *The Methuselah Factor Diet and Lifestyle Program*.)

However, we didn't stop there. We included data from a German study that looked at another hemorheology-enhancing practice: blood donation.[40] Berlin-based researcher Sundrela Kamhieh-Milz and colleagues studied 146 people with elevated blood pressures who donated blood four times over the course of a year. The blood donors logged striking benefits: their systolic readings (the upper blood pressure value) dropped an average of 12.2 points while their diastolic numbers fell 6.9 points.

By now, you've probably guessed: blood donation is another recommended practice in *The Methuselah Factor Diet and Lifestyle Program*.

Clearly, the medical evidence adds high blood pressure to our list of Methuselah-Factor-related conditions. The message is clear:

if you have high blood pressure, then you need to improve your blood fluidity. *The Methuselah Factor Diet and Lifestyle Program* is tailored to fit your needs. And if you *must* do something before diving whole heartedly into the program, why not find out where your local blood bank is—and start getting yourself psyched up to be a blood donor.

9

IMPROVE YOUR METHUSELAH FACTOR, HELP AVOID DIABETES AND ITS COMPLICATIONS

DIABETES CONSTITUTES ONE OF the world's great epidemics. Rates of diabetes throughout the world are surging. I can remember lecturing on diabetes in the 1990s. A well accepted statistic at that time was that 800,000 new cases were being diagnosed each year in the U.S. If that sounds dizzying, hold on. Currently, newly diagnosed diabetes cases number 1.5 million annually.[41] However, the U.S. is the tip of the iceberg. The World Health Organization recently stated that 422 million adults were currently living with diabetes, nearly a four-fold rise from the 108 million affected in 1980.[42]

Diabetes brings us to another chapter in our search for connections between the Methuselah Factor and disease. We have been looking at factors that influence hemorheology in isolation, such as white blood cell count, fibrinogen levels, and platelets.

However, we haven't really looked at something that can raise levels of all these Methuselah Factor components: inflammation.

To understand these connections, we need to quickly review the diabetic process. Most lay people think of diabetes as a problem due to insufficient insulin production. There's some truth in that, but it largely misses the most important aspects of the cause and treatment of *most* cases.

Type 1 diabetes is responsible for a relatively small percentage (5-10%) of the diabetes cases in America. In this condition, as manifested in what we used to call "juvenile diabetes," the root cause is, indeed, insufficient insulin production. Most cases of type 1 diabetes, whether in childhood or adulthood (yes, this type of diabetes can, uncommonly, affect adults), is typically caused by an autoimmune process. Foreign proteins (antigens)—such as those introduced by certain viruses—appear to trigger an overly aggressive immune response. Casualties in that immune warfare are the insulin-producing islet cells (beta cells) of the pancreas. At this point, other than receiving a transplanted pancreas—or transplanted islet cells—type 1 diabetes is an irreversible disease. Lifelong insulin therapy is necessary.

In sharp distinction to type 1 diabetes stands the type 2 variety (accounting for 90-95% of cases in America, and the majority of cases worldwide[43,44]). Formerly called "adult-onset diabetes," type 2 has a totally different root cause; namely, insulin resistance. (The adult-onset moniker no longer fits: not only can adults be afflicted with type 1 diabetes, but also more and more children are being diagnosed with what we used to call this adult onset variety.)

What is insulin resistance? It is simply insulin not working as it should. Normally insulin "opens doors" in your cells that allow sugar to leave your bloodstream and enter into your tissues, where it is used for fuel. Consequently, we could personify insulin as the doorman who opens those vital doors. Insulin resistance would then be analogous to "gummed up" doors, or doors with rusted hinges. For the sake of our metaphor, these damaged doors, now extremely difficult to open, require more than one doorman to pry them ajar and allow the blood sugar to get into your cells. What does your body do? Your pancreas sends more doormen/insulin to each cell to get the job done.

Don't miss this point. In typical type 2 diabetes, before you ever get this condition, your pancreas is making more insulin than normal, attempting to overcome the effects of insulin resistance. In fact, many newly-diagnosed individuals with diabetes have blood insulin levels markedly higher than their average non-diabetic neighbors.[45]

Unfortunately, if the insulin resistant state is not addressed, it tends to inexorably worsen. For many, the time comes when their pancreas can no longer keep churning out huge amounts of insulin. The result? Not enough doormen to open those insulin-resistant doors. Sufficient amounts of sugar can't get into the cells. Blood sugar rises. Diabetes is diagnosed.

Now let's review. Ninety to ninety-five percent of diabetes in America is of the type 2 variety. And the root cause of this form of diabetes is insulin resistance. Now here's where the good news comes in. Insulin resistance is, largely, reversible. That's right: address the underlying causes of the insulin resistant state and a person's diabetes may go into remission.

This is not conjecture. I've seen it with my own eyes hundreds of times. Over the years, I've worked in centers using state-of-the art natural and lifestyle strategies to reverse insulin resistance. I've seen many patients with type 2 diabetes throw away their insulin and actually have better blood sugars. I've seen many patients on oral medications for their type 2 diabetes either decrease or eliminate their pills—and have better blood sugars.

Remember, we're talking only type 2 diabetes, not type 1. The message: address insulin resistance, and thus help reverse the diabetic state.

Now here's where the Methuselah Factor comes in. Poorer blood fluidity is connected to insulin resistance—independent of diabetes. How do we know this? One answer comes from understanding a condition caused by insulin resistance, whether or not diabetes is present. It is called the Metabolic Syndrome.

When individuals with this syndrome are studied, they invariably have less than optimal hemorheology. Note in Figure 9 that among the hemorheology-impairing factors mentioned is "inflammation."[46,47,48,49,50,51] Although inflammatory processes can be triggered by trauma, surgery, infections or other diseases, lifestyle can also trigger inflammation—and with that inflammation comes worsened blood fluidity and an increased risk of diabetes. When we carry extra weight, especially around our midsection, fat cells themselves pump out inflammation-boosting compounds.

Now we're faced with the chicken-or-egg question. Does the metabolic syndrome cause Methuselah Factor abnormalities, or do the Methuselah Factor defects tend to foster insulin resistance— and its consequences like diabetes and the metabolic syndrome? The evidence seems to suggest both are true. Insulin resistance impairs hemorheology, but poor hemorheology also worsens insulin resistance. One medical monograph connected some of the dots in this way: "Microvascular dysfunction [i.e., unhealthy tiny blood vessels that don't relax properly], by affecting both flow resistance and tissue perfusion, seems important… in the development of hypertension and insulin resistance."[52]

In short, if you decrease blood supply to your tissues, then your

FIGURE 9 Insulin Resistance and the
Methuselah Factor

Even without diabetes, higher than optimal insulin
levels (a sign of insulin resistance such as seen in the
metabolic syndrome) increase RBC aggregation
which, in turn, impairs optimal circulation.[46]

The more insulin resistance a person has, the worse his
or her blood fluidity. This fact has been indicated by
markers such as higher plasma viscosity readings,
elevated fibrinogen levels, and increased
hematocrit.[47, 48, 49]

Inflammatory processes — such as those triggered by
carrying extra weight — raise levels of compounds that
worsen blood fluidity like white blood cell count and
fibrinogen; these in turn, are linked to greater insulin
resistance and/or increased risk of developing
diabetes.[50, 51]

insulin resistance will worsen. This would be expected, regardless
of the cause of the impaired circulation. Additional evidence bol-
sters this claim. A variety of studies from around the world indicate that factors that worsen blood fluidity are associated with
worsened insulin resistance.[53]

Why would poor tissue blood supply (resulting from less than
desirable hemorheology) be linked to insulin resistance? The situation is analogous to that with high blood pressure. Remember
the relationship: worsen blood flow in your small blood vessels,
decrease oxygen delivery to the blood-vessel-lining endothelial cells, add to their "oxidative stress," and impair their relaxant

function. When you realize oxidative stress worsens insulin resistance, the picture is complete.

Consider another line of evidence. Even if impaired hemorheology is not your problem, other things might decrease oxygen delivery to your tissues. If what we have been saying is true, then insulin resistance would increase in these other settings of deficient tissue oxygenation. This is exactly what the research shows. For example, two groups whose tissues get less oxygen are (1) individuals with serious respiratory disease and (2) physically fit mountain climbers at high elevation. You guessed it. Both groups experience increased insulin resistance.[54,55]

But there's more. To do its job, insulin has to get to the site of action. The doorman can't open the doors if he's not there. So, if your blood fluidity is impaired, you won't be able to get optimal amounts of insulin to your tissues.[56]

If all this is not convincing enough, consider yet another piece of evidence linking poor tissue blood flow with the development of diabetes. Granted, this study did not look at the Methuselah Factor per se; it looked, instead, at permanent narrowing of tiny blood *vessels in the only place where we can directly visualize them*, in the retina of the eye. (Yes, that's one of the things your eye doctor is looking at when she uses that fancy instrument called a slit lamp to look through your eye's natural lens to the very back of your eye.)

Dr. Tien Yin Wong and colleagues analyzed data from the U.S. Atherosclerosis Risk in Communities Study.[57] This large study involved nearly 8000 individuals aged 49 to 73 years who were initially diabetes-free. At the outset of this particular investigation, the researchers measured the size of the tiny arteries in each subject's retina. The specific measurement that they recorded is called the A:V ratio, a comparison between the size of the arteries in relation to the veins. (If small arteries are exposed to unhealthy situations, their diameter tends to decrease relative to the veins).

Wong and collaborators then followed this population for about 3.5 years, diagnosing nearly 300 new cases of diabetes in the process. Figure 10 shows their remarkable findings—especially when you realize that changes in eye blood vessels reflect what is happening in all the small blood vessels throughout the body. The implications seem clear: impair circulation in your tiny blood vessels, increase your risk of developing diabetes.

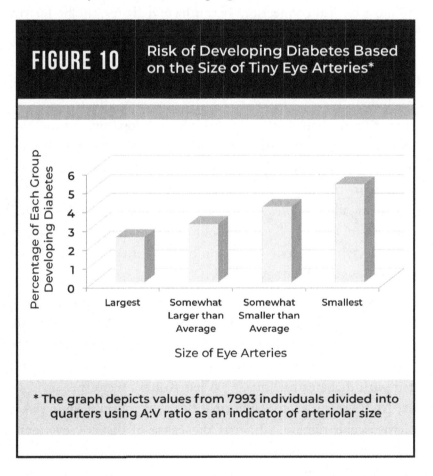

FIGURE 10 Risk of Developing Diabetes Based on the Size of Tiny Eye Arteries*

* The graph depicts values from 7993 individuals divided into quarters using A:V ratio as an indicator of arteriolar size

Some naysayers, nevertheless, will insist that the only connection between insulin resistance and impaired hemorheology is that the former causes the latter. Of course, I think that the research convincingly suggests otherwise. But let's concede the point. If a bad Methuselah Factor doesn't help set the stage for insulin resistance, can people with diabetes just shelve this book once and for all?

Quite the contrary. There's much more to the relationship between the Methuselah Factor and diabetes. Here's perhaps the most critical connection: if you have diabetes, the better your blood fluidity, the less your risk of diabetic complications.

In a review of the scientific literature on this topic, Dr. Young Cho from Philadelphia's Drexel University and his collaborators concluded: "increased blood viscosity adversely affects the microcirculation in diabetes, leading to microangiopathy."[58] Lay translation: diabetes worsens the Methuselah Factor (by adversely impacting things like blood viscosity). This, in turn, worsens circulation in the tiny blood vessels, leading to "microangiopathy," i.e., the small blood vessel complications of diabetes. These small blood vessel changes lie at the root of many of diabetes' common side effects: blindness, nerve problems (often contributing to amputations), and kidney failure.

Katalin Koltai and colleagues at The University of Pecs School of Medicine in Hungary went a step further: "Rheological factors and increased platelet aggregation are convincingly implicated in the development of micro- and macrovascular disease associated with diabetes mellitus."[59] What Koltai's team was saying is: yes, Methuselah Factor abnormalities will increase your risk of microvascular disease, which is the cause of diabetic eye, nerve, and kidney complications. However, poor hemorheology will also up your chances of succumbing to the macrovascular (large vessel) complications of diabetes. These are the complications that increase the risk of diabetes-related killers like heart attack and stroke.

The practical messages are twofold. First, type 2 diabetes, in many cases, is reversible by following a diet and lifestyle that addresses blood fluidity. Second, if you have diabetes—type 1 or 2—you likely can decrease your risk of complications by paying heed to hemorheology.

10

IMPROVE YOUR METHUSELAH FACTOR, GET HELP FOR SHEDDING EXCESS POUNDS

TALLY UP ALL THE weight-loss classes, slim-down self-help books, body-fat trimming medications, and bariatric surgeries and you end up with a $66 billion annual industry in the United States.[60] However, that's only a fraction of costs associated with our expanding waistlines. All told, the United States Centers for Disease Control and Prevention puts the price tag for overweight and obesity at over $150 billion per year.[61]

Furthermore, this year some 100 million of us will try to shed pounds by dieting alone. In other words, if you're an American, there's a good chance you're either reading this book as part of a plan to slim down or you'll be taking such steps—with or without this book—sometime over the next 12 months.

In view of the huge price tag, the numbers affected, and the often drastic measures employed to lose weight, is it possible that something as simple as improving your blood fluidity could play a key role in helping you finally gain control over your waistline?

The surprising answer—at least to the uninitiated—is "yes." (But, after all we've learned so far about the Methuselah Factor, this insight probably didn't take *you* unawares.)

So, what's the evidence for the hemorheology-weight gain connection?

One of the more interesting studies that shed light on this relationship appeared in 2000 in the journal *Obesity Research*. There, Bruce Duncan and colleagues reported on some fascinating insights gained from the Atherosclerosis Risk in Communities (ARIC) study. This large study, involving 13,017 men and women, 45 to 64 years of age, yielded some fascinating insights about body weight.

Specifically, Duncan and his team looked to see if subjects with evidence of worse hemorheology were more likely to gain weight than those with better blood fluidity over a relatively short, three-year period. In order to do this, the researchers honed in on individuals who gained a significant amount of weight (i.e., were in the upper 10% of weight gainers) during that time frame. Then they used something called "interquartile comparisons" to see if those in the worst quarter of the population for various Methuselah Factor components were more likely to be among the big gainers. This is exactly what they found, as illustrated in Figure 11.

As indicated by the graphic, individuals whose fibrinogen levels were in the top 25% were 60% more likely to gain a substantial amount of weight compared to those with fibrinogen levels in the lower quarter. The same relative relationships held true with other markers of the Methuselah Factor, like white blood cell count (WBC) and von Willebrand factor. Having higher values appeared to put individuals at greater risk of weight gain. (Factor VIII is another blood clotting protein where higher levels indicate worse blood fluidity.)

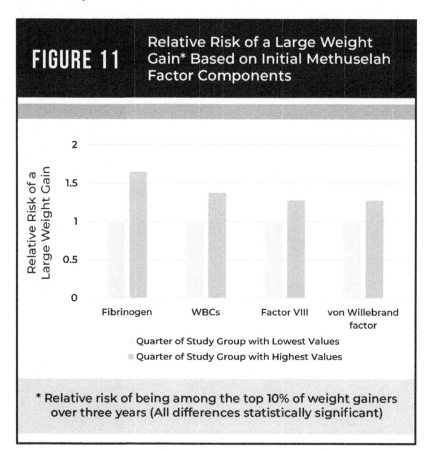

FIGURE 11 Relative Risk of a Large Weight Gain* Based on Initial Methuselah Factor Components

* Relative risk of being among the top 10% of weight gainers over three years (All differences statistically significant)

Why would poor blood fluidity increase your risk of weight problems? One explanation for the relationship is this: poor hemorheology impairs optimal tissue oxygenation, and when tissue oxygen delivery suffers, your metabolism slows. Slower metabolism, in turn, puts you at greater risk of weight gain. Consequently, the data suggests a powerful, yet overlooked weight-loss key: improve your Methuselah Factor.

11

IMPROVE YOUR METHUSELAH FACTOR, IMPROVE YOUR BONE AND JOINT HEALTH

WE LIVE IN AN age of tremendous medical progress. Many orthopedic problems that crippled our forefathers have now loosened their hold on quality of life because of technologies like arthroscopic surgery and joint replacement.

Although you no doubt know firsthand of individuals (perhaps yourself) who are living testimonies to the blessings of an artificial knee or hip, orthopedic issues still rank as major causes of pain and suffering.

I would not presume to say that the Methuselah Factor is related to every bone or joint condition. However, there is compelling evidence that at least some of our most disabling orthopedic problems could be helped or prevented by improving blood fluidity.

Autoimmune diseases like lupus and rheumatoid arthritis (RA) are known to be associated with blood fluidity impairments. Many doctors again go down that same chicken-or-the-egg path they did with diabetes. However, such discussions seem moot when it comes to these autoimmune forms of arthritis.

Here's why. *The Methuselah Factor Diet and Lifestyle Program* seems calculated to help many individuals with lupus, RA, and similar disorders. Whether or not that help is derived wholly, in part, or not at all from improved blood fluidity is immaterial when you consider two things. First, lifestyle habits that tend to improve hemorheology tend to help these autoimmune conditions.[62] Second, some of the ravages of these diseases can be decreased by paying attention to blood fluidity.[63] Researchers are suggesting that a growing body of evidence indicates a connection between these so called "collagen vascular diseases" and poor blood rheology. Improving blood fluidity may thus help a host of autoimmune rheumatologic conditions.[64]

A growing body of literature suggests an even more common cause of orthopedic pain and suffering is related, at least in part, to impaired circulation. That problem is chronic back pain.

In the United States, during any given 3-month span, the data suggests that 28% of adults will have to deal with painful low back problems.[65] These conditions, which can be chronic, are a major cause of orthopedic limitations. Medical research has now drawn some interesting connections between back problems and poor blood fluidity.

After reviewing nearly 200 medical studies, Finnish researcher, L.I. Kauppila concluded there was a connection between disordered blood flow to the spine and both low back pain and degenerative disc disease (DDD).[66] Degenerative disc disease affects the integrity of the cushioning elements between the bones of your back. (See Figure 12.) It can contribute to herniated or bulging discs, which can put pressure on the spinal cord and/or nerves.

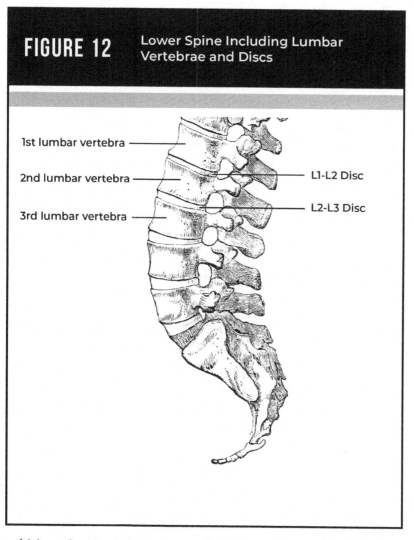

FIGURE 12 — Lower Spine Including Lumbar Vertebrae and Discs

1st lumbar vertebra

2nd lumbar vertebra

3rd lumbar vertebra

L1-L2 Disc

L2-L3 Disc

Although most of the research has been focused on blockage in the larger arteries supplying the back (rather than on hemorheology and microcirculation), a couple of observations are relevant. First, we have already seen that blockages in large blood vessels (such as those supplying the heart and brain) are linked to poor hemorheology. Thus, the Methuselah Factor is also involved in low back circulation. Second, data is now linking risk of heart disease with risk of low back problems—and that linkage may not be explained by conventional heart disease risk factors like high cholesterol, cigarette smoking, or elevated blood pressure.[67] Might poor hemorheology be a better explanation? Further research is needed.

Let's look at one other area where connections are emerging between hemorheology and joint problems: knee osteoarthritis (OA). If you're not familiar with the terminology, *osteoarthritis* refers to the most common form of arthritis, believed to be caused by cumulative wear and tear on the joints. It is also referred to as degenerative joint disease.

Our knees are among the most common places to experience disabling complications from osteoarthritis. What are we learning about OA of our knees?

Years before the onset of OA, we can assess the health of our knees, and their risk of long-term arthritis, by measuring something called "tibial cartilage volume." Such an assessment evaluates how much cushioning surface (cartilage) overlies the tibia, the largest bone in our lower legs, which provides the lower boundary of the knee joint. Simply put, as one group of researchers recently described it, "In a young adult without OA, tibial cartilage volume is a measure of knee joint health."[68] However, these investigators were not content to just review current medical research. When studying a representative sample of adult men and women from Australia (mean age 35), the research team made a remarkable discovery. Indicators of poor hemorheology, like fibrinogen, were associated with less tibial cartilage. Although high fibrinogen levels may be markers of inflammation or obesity, the observation is still intriguing. It adds just one more piece of evidence to the possibility that poor hemorheology increases our risk for joint problems, while Methuselah Factor improvement is good for our joints.

If you manage to live without arthritis, there's a good chance you'll deal with another bone health condition: osteoporosis. Although being overweight increases our risk for arthritis, it actually decreases our risk of osteoporosis or thinning of the bones. So, in a very real sense, our body composition puts us at risk for one or the other of these disorders.

The good news is this: evidence is accumulating that improving our Methuselah Factor might help us avoid osteoporosis.[69] This is not surprising. If our microcirculation is not healthy, our bone health—just like our joint health—might suffer. Further strengthening these observations is a connection between osteoporosis and heart disease, possibly both due to effects of poor blood fluidity.[70]

It's not a slam dunk case. But if you have arthritic problems or osteoporosis, the data suggests that attention to the Methuselah Factor might help you improve the health of your bones and joints.

12

IMPROVE YOUR METHUSELAH FACTOR, DELAY AGING

ONE OF THE GREATEST fears associated with aging is cognitive decline. Fortunately, we have already noted that improved hemorheology appears calculated to improve our mental functioning. But what about our physical abilities? Can better blood fluidity help slow the physical decline that often occurs with time?

The answer may seem obvious. After all, if our physical health declines during our "golden" years, likely implicated is one or more of the conditions we've already found linked to the Methuselah Factor. If it's not vision problems, arthritis, diabetes, or the ravages of circulatory disorders that make us feel like "we're getting old," then what is?

However, the medical research gives evidence of some profound relationships that transcend such theoretical generalities. Figure 13 lists some of the documented changes in blood fluidity that tend to accompany aging.[71,72,73,74,75,76,77]

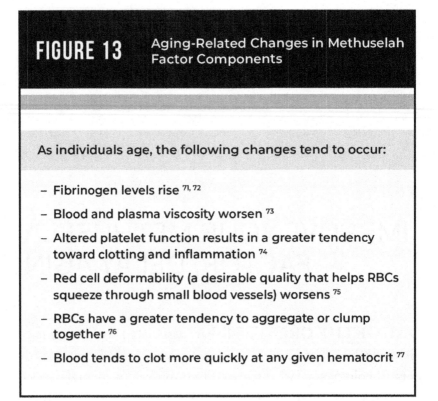

FIGURE 13   Aging-Related Changes in Methuselah Factor Components

As individuals age, the following changes tend to occur:

- Fibrinogen levels rise [71, 72]

- Blood and plasma viscosity worsen [73]

- Altered platelet function results in a greater tendency toward clotting and inflammation [74]

- Red cell deformability (a desirable quality that helps RBCs squeeze through small blood vessels) worsens [75]

- RBCs have a greater tendency to aggregate or clump together [76]

- Blood tends to clot more quickly at any given hematocrit [77]

In view of the myriad Methuselah Factor abnormalities that seem to creep up on us as we age, strategies to improve hemorheology stand calculated to help undo some of time's physical ravages. Preliminary data suggests that diet and other lifestyle practices may have a role in slowing—or reversing—these age-related changes.[78]

Granted, there is much we still do not know. Aging, with its associated decrements in hemorheology and increases in inflammation, continues to be fertile ground for research. However, the state of the science at this point suggests that both Methuselah Factor impairments and inflammation drive some of aging's consequences—both physical and mental.

Illustrative of these connections, research from the University of Florida suggested that Methuselah-Factor-worsening blood characteristics like activated platelets could contribute to mobility limitations that commonly occur with aging.[79] Subsequently, a team of South Korean researchers studied 57 non-obese, middle-aged men (34-55 years old), for three years. They documented age-related changes that contributed to inflammation and impaired blood flow (in this case, resulting from increased arterial stiffness).[80]

Existing research connects aging with increased inflammation, worsened hemorheology, and poorer blood flow. Although there are still many unanswered questions, we don't need to wait until all the answers are in. Regardless of how young we think we are, to some extent we are all in a race against the clock. The evidence from the aging literature suggests that each of us need to get serious *today* about improving our Methuselah Factor. This gives us the best chance of maintaining our current physical capacities for as long as possible.

13

IMPROVE YOUR METHUSELAH FACTOR, IMPROVE PHYSICAL PERFORMANCE

EARLIER IN THIS BOOK we studied how elite athletes have engaged in blood doping, a hemorheology-impairing behavior that actually improves athletic performance. In communicating that information, I realized some may have concluded that improving one's Methuselah Factor is important if you are old and/or diseased, but if you are young and healthy, you just may have to worsen your blood fluidity in order to perform better.

As compelling as that logic might sound, it is generally false. Granted, one Methuselah Factor-impairing component is associated with better performance, namely, a higher hematocrit. However, other blood fluidity considerations could be summarized simply: improve your Methuselah Factor and you will improve your performance.

Consider a few examples. In 2009, French researchers gave athletes an antioxidant supplement. As we have already alluded to (and will see further in upcoming chapters), boosting one's antioxidant status is almost a guarantee of improving one's hemorheology. For years, the medical literature has suggested Methuselah Factor benefits when athletes supplement with antioxidants.[81] Well, what else do you think happens when athletes improve their dietary antioxidant status? No surprises. They significantly improve their performance.[82]

Although other studies have questioned the benefits of aggressive antioxidant supplementation—because stress on the body is what helps athletes get more fit as they train—the provocative connection remains.[83,84] Improving the Methuselah Factor seems to correlate with better performance.

European researcher J.F. Brun and colleagues have studied rugby players—both male and female—over the past several decades.[85,86] They found impressive connections between poorer blood fluidity and poorer athletic performance as summarized in Figure 14.

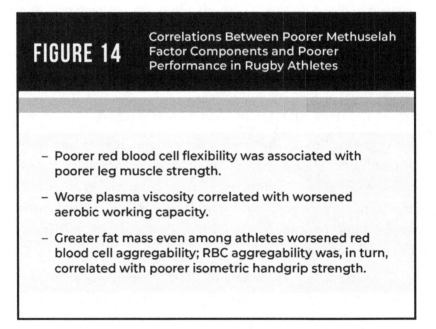

FIGURE 14 — Correlations Between Poorer Methuselah Factor Components and Poorer Performance in Rugby Athletes

– Poorer red blood cell flexibility was associated with poorer leg muscle strength.

– Worse plasma viscosity correlated with worsened aerobic working capacity.

– Greater fat mass even among athletes worsened red blood cell aggregability; RBC aggregability was, in turn, correlated with poorer isometric handgrip strength.

Bottom line: even if you are healthy and fit, an emphasis on hemorheology can improve your physical performance—in addition to the cognitive benefits we noted earlier. *The Methuselah Factor Diet and Lifestyle* is relevant for you as well.

Time to Act

As we have seen, medical scientists are realizing that the Methuselah Factor, hemorheology, is incredibly important, influencing a growing number of disease states—and helping us optimize physical and mental performance at any age. That's why more voices are clamoring to include hemorheology measurements as part of standard laboratory evaluations.[87]

The day may not be far off when your doctor routinely measures your blood viscosity or other Methuselah Factor markers. However, we don't need to wait until then to reap the benefits of better blood fluidity.

With our minds sensitized to the importance of hemorheology, we're now ready to embark on our thirty-day journey to improve your blood fluidity through *The Methuselah Factor Diet and Lifestyle Program*.

Part 2

DAY BY DAY, THE THIRTY-DAY METHUSELAH FACTOR DIET AND LIFESTYLE PROGRAM

14

GET READY, GET SET...

REGARDLESS OF HOW DEEPLY you immersed yourself into the science behind Chapters 3 to 13, you're likely beginning to sense how a skillful application of Methuselah Factor principles can help elevate your health to a new level. We're now ready to embark on our thirty-day journey toward a longer, healthier and, yes, better life.

In Chapter 2, I gave you an overview of how *The Methuselah Factor Diet and Lifestyle Program* works. However, I now need to provide a review along with some additional details.

The Program will evolve over the course of the next thirty chapters. In general, each chapter focuses on a specific lifestyle challenge to be implemented over the course of the thirty-day program. I might call on you to adopt a new lifestyle practice or recommit to something good you're already doing.

Figure 15 puts those upcoming chapters into a table format that you will use to record your goals—and chart your progress.

Chapt # (Day #)	15 (1)	16 (2)	17 (3)	18 (4)	19 (5)	20 (6)	21 (7)	22 (8)	23 (9)	24 (10)	25 (11)	26 (12)	27 (13)	28 (14)	29 (15)
Day #	Call a local blood bank	Measure ___ times per day/week	Get ___ min exercise per day/week	Eat beans daily	Daily connect with someone about this program	Only have ___ caffeinated drinks per day/week	Set aside one day for rest weekly	Decrease salt consumption	Do resistance exercise ___ times per week	Go meat-free ___ days per week	Follow at least two healthy sleep principles nightly	Drink ___ ounces of water per day	Use hydrotherapy at least once per week	Focus on spiritual health during your weekly rest day	I will daily ___ to help me lose weight
1															
2															
3															
4															
5															
6															
7															
Wk 1 Total															
9															
10															
11															
12															
13															
14															
Wk 2 Total															
15															
16															
17															
18															
19															
20															
21															
Wk 3 Total															
22															
23															
24															
25															
26															
27															
28															
Wk 4 Total															
29															
30															

Chapt # (Day #)	30 (16) Do daily deep breathing exercises	31 (17) Avoid high-sugar foods	32 (18) Implement this environmental strategy:	33 (19) Increase green vegetable intake daily OR do a vegetable fast one day per week	34 (20) Improve daily oral care OR increase your daily intake of magnesium	35 (21) Improve at least one of your previous target behaviors	36 (22) Engage in some type of fasting either daily or weekly	37 (23) Fill out Figure 19	38 (24) Eliminate the following stressor:	39 (25) Implement a strategy to harness this stressor:	40 (26) Eliminate any supplements that are neither prescribed nor of clear benefit	41 (27) To my daily regimen, add the following supplement:	42 (28) Forgive _____ OR perform one act of unmerited kindness daily	43 (29) Boost melatonin with lifestyle practices OR take a melatonin supplement	44 (30) Stick with at least one of your new lifestyle habits for 30 more days
Day #															
16															
17															
18															
19															
20															
21															
Wk 3 Total															
22															
23															
24															
25															
26															
27															
28															
Wk 4 Total															
29															
30															

There's really no substitute for Figure 15 to keep yourself accountable—and on target. (Some of the text in Figure 15 appears in fine print. If you would like a larger version, you can download it for free at: www.compasshealth.net/figure-15.) Now, here's how Figure 15 works.

The first row in Figure 15 identifies each day of the program and its corresponding chapter in this book. The next row walks you through each of the succeeding chapters of this book. For example, the next chapter (Chapter 15) is entitled "Be Bold, Call the Bank." That chapter gives you some marching orders for the entire thirty days (encouraging you to set lofty behavioral goals rather than taking the path of least resistance for a month). However, it also challenges you to put in a single call to your local blood bank. Once you've done that simple task, with each passing day, you'll be able to check off that first column. For example, if you call the blood bank on the third day of your program, then on each subsequent day (Days 4 to 30) you'll get to put an "X" in that column. It was a one-time challenge, so you've accomplished that goal for the entire program.

Of course, the cells for Days 1 and 2 in that column will remain blank (unchecked) because you had not yet made the phone call on either of those days. (Note: the one-time goal for Day 1 is unique. Every subsequent day of the program you will be committed to something that you have to do with some recurring frequency during the thirty days.)

Now look back at the top two rows on the chart. The next column focuses on Chapter 16 and Day 2 of your program. You can probably correctly surmise that the challenge on that day will be to decide *what to measure* and *at what frequency* throughout the course of your thirty-day program. If you are overweight, you may commit to "weighing in" once a week. If you're dealing with high blood pressure, then you might set a goal of taking your BP twice daily. If you have diabetes, your commitment might involve checking your blood sugar three times per day. In that latter scenario, you would fill in the blanks as follows: *measure* blood sugar, 3 *times per day/week.* Then circle "day" to indicate you're setting a daily, as opposed to a weekly goal.

Note that not every cell in the second row (the row right below the chapter numbers) has something for you to fill in. However, because of the program's flexibility, you'll have to finalize *some* of the details on *some* of the days. Of course, Figure 15 is not designed to be filled out at a single sitting. Each day you'll read the relevant chapter. Upon completing the chapter, you will make a specific new commitment. If that commitment requires some fine-tuning on your end, you'll then add those personalized details to the second row. And, of course, that goal will be one that you will continue to follow for the rest of the thirty days.

The remainder of the rows in Figure 15 are designed to chart your daily progress with respect to each of your goals. We have already seen that under the *row* for Day 1 (i.e., the third row from the top of the table) you will either put a check mark indicating that you called the blood bank, or you'll leave the box blank (or filled with a zero) if you haven't. However, when you come to the next row, for Day 2 (i.e., the fourth row from the top of the table), you'll first indicate whether or not you've called the blood bank, and then you'll move to the next column where you'll indicate the number of times you checked your blood sugar that day. You can write in the number "3" if you met your goal of three blood sugar checks daily, or you could simply mark an "X" for reaching your goal. (I prefer the former method of charting as it lets you better visualize your progress.)

Some readers may bristle at the idea of a checklist, especially one that you have to use every day of the thirty-day program. However, just think back on your last commercial airline flight.

You obviously survived the experience; you're reading this book. But one of the reasons you survived is this: the flight crew completed their checklists. In the airline industry those checklists are designed to ensure that nothing is overlooked when it comes to getting the passengers safely to their destination.

It is the same with *The Methuselah Factor Diet and Lifestyle Program*. Figure 15 is essential to keep us all on track. And it is really not all that onerous. Only on Day 30 are there actually thirty things to track. And most all of the activities are things that can be charted in a moment—especially if you make a point to be attentive to your daily lifestyle choices. Also remember: I'm asking you to follow the comprehensive plan *only* for thirty days.

I'll be the first to admit that the diet gurus now have grounds to tar and feather me. They'll argue that any temporary plan will not yield long-term results. They're right—and they're wrong. Let me explain.

If you follow *The Methuselah Factor Diet and Lifestyle* for thirty days only, and then go totally back to your old way of living, you really are not likely to gain—or lose (in the case of weight)—much. True, over the course of your one-month journey, you may feel a bit better, sleep more soundly, and trim down somewhat. However, if you fully retreat to your old lifestyle after the thirty days, those benefits will most likely evaporate quickly.

But here's where the experts are wrong. *The Methuselah Factor Diet and Lifestyle* is so powerful that most of you will never return, at least completely, to your old way of living. I've worked with patients for some three decades implementing intensive lifestyle change programs that utilize the Methuselah Factor principles. An illustrative response was expressed years ago by Hector, one of our patients: "When I started, I had no intention of following this program long term. However, seeing how much progress I've made, I'd be a fool to not continue this entire program for the rest of my life."

This is where Figure 16 comes in, where you track your personal improvements—not just lifestyle changes. Now I realize that Figure 16 might seem a lot like the column for Chapter 16 (Day 2) in Figure 15. However, in Figure 16, you try to track a variety of biological markers over the course of the program. Some of you may want to collect some of these values only at the very beginning and ending of your program (like the various blood measurements). For many of you it won't make much sense to list these as goals in Figure 15. In other words, save the column for Day 2 in Figure 15 to indicate measurements you will make on a daily or weekly basis. With Figure 16, no matter what your personal goals are, try to obtain each of the measurements listed, at least at the start and finish of your program.[88]

As you read through each of the subsequent chapters, one per day, you will be given fresh assignments to follow for the rest of your month-long journey. Keep tables 15 and 16 bookmarked. Refer to them, daily. Each daily assignment will keep you focused. Visual reminders of your progress will, yes, keep you motivated.

If you're ready to begin the thirty-day journey today, great. Read the next chapter and begin filling out Figure 15. If your start date is still a few days off, that's fine. However, once you start on your journey, be faithful. Read just one chapter per day. Accept each of the daily challenges, choosing a strategy that you can fit into your lifestyle. Continue those behaviors for the thirty days and you'll likely be surprised by how much progress you will make over the course of the month.

FIGURE 16

Personal Improvements While Following the 30-Day Program

End of Week #	Weight	Fasting Blood Sugar	HgbA1c (average blood sugar test)	Blood Pressure	Total Cholesetrol (fasting)
0 (before you start the program)					
1					
2					
3					
4					
5 (one to five days after program completion)					

FIGURE 16
(CONTINUED)

Personal Improvements While Following the 30-Day Program

End of Week #	LDL Cholesterol (fasting)	HDL Cholesterol (fasting)	Triglycerides (fasting)	Other Improvements
0 (before you start the program)				
1				
2				
3				
4				
5 (one to five days after program completion)				

15

DAY 1: BE BOLD; CALL THE BANK

Today's Challenge: Determine to set significant personal goals each day of this thirty-day program. Start by making a call to your local blood bank.

I STILL REMEMBER IT well, growing up in the DeRose household. My parents really wanted the best for me. Therefore, it wasn't uncommon at dinner time to find some green leafy vegetables on my plate.

Now I must admit, leafy greens were not my favorite childhood food. As a result, I was often doing well just to be using my fork to move those green leafy vegetables around on my plate. But, sooner or later, I'd get a message from my dad that went something like this: "David, eat those greens. They're good for you."

I didn't realize it at the time, but a connection was developing in my brain: *tastes bad, good for me*. If that illustration sounds familiar, it's one that I've shared with live audiences for many years. It also made its way into my popular DVD series: *Changing Bad Habits for Good.*

However, throughout my childhood I was making other connections. I recall often being told that things I enjoyed, like cookies or candy—especially at odd hours—were unhealthy. Yes, another connection that developed in my young brain was *tastes good, bad for me.*

As I've dealt with patients and audiences, I found that many of us grew up with these very same connections. We emerged from childhood with the idea that somehow the things we find most enjoyable are typically not healthy, while the *healthy* items are ones generally unpalatable.

As a result, we develop a mental dichotomy. We think that one of our life tasks is to decide whether we want to be happy or whether, instead, we prefer to be healthy. Or, more likely, how much ill-health we can tolerate in order to make life sufficiently enjoyable. Fortunately, this dichotomy is false. Medical research indicates that the very habits that help us live longer are the same ones that add quality to our lives.

One place this is seen clearly is in the science of hemorheology. After all, the Methuselah Factor helps us with things that we normally put in the physical health realm like avoiding heart attacks, strokes, and cancer. However, we've seen that improved blood fluidity also increases our likelihood of having a happy life by impacting things like our mental clarity, our sense of wellbeing, and our physical performance.

Each of us has an amazing ability to develop new enjoyments. I've been reminded of this many times in talking with cigarette-smoking patients. If I ask one about his or her very first smoke, invariably I'll hear a story of coughing, nausea, and perhaps even vomiting.

How could anyone get hooked on something that their body initially found so repulsive? Simply by persistence. Yes, nicotine was there to provide an addictive hook. However, the fact remains: millions of people on the globe have taken up habits that they initially found repulsive, but now enjoy.

This dynamic works not only with addictions and what we typically label as *bad habits*. It works with good habits as well. When we wrote our best-selling book, *Thirty Days to Natural Blood Pressure Control*, we shared classic research published some three decades ago that focused on sodium intake. Christina Blais and colleagues at the University of Minnesota found that subjects who drastically cut their salt intake ended up enjoying foods substantially less salty.[89] After three months, those study participants preferred soups with half as much salt.

My challenge to you the first day of this new program? Be Bold. Since you no longer need to fear that you'll have to give up happiness to be healthy, you're free to ask another question: *What's the healthiest lifestyle for which I can develop an enjoyment?* I would like to suggest such a lifestyle will seek to optimize your Methuselah Factor.

So, *be bold* as you look at each day's assignment. Don't ask how little you can do but, rather, ask yourself what bold changes you can make to further improve your blood fluidity.

Each day of our thirty-day journey, I'm asking you to put away your preconceived ideas. Determine to try something new for the rest of the month. And don't forget to keep your healthcare provider in the loop. I'm along on this journey as a fellow traveler and educator. I'm not your doctor. Let your primary care provider know your plans and keep in touch with his or her office so that they can help you keep an eye out for any changes. For example, on a blood-fluidity-optimizing program, such as the one found in these pages, you should expect significant improvement in disease processes like high blood pressure and diabetes. Therefore, if you're on medications for your pressure or sugar, there's a good chance you'll have to work with your doctor to decrease those medications.

Now, I promised you a challenge every day. Specifically, I told you I would give you something *to do* each day that would move you in the direction of better hemorheology.

So, although *being bold* might be a rallying cry for the entire book, it's hardly a specific challenge. That's where the second part of this chapter's title comes from: *Call the Bank.*

As you should know, I'm not asking you to contact a financial institution or to put any money on the line. Instead, your challenge in this chapter is to call your local *blood bank.*

Why? Medical research reveals that hemorheology significantly improves following blood donation. This is illustrated by measurements of blood viscosity following the donation of even a single pint of blood.[90] The clinical benefits of donation were practically illustrated earlier when we focused on the research of Dr. Kamhieh-Milz and associates. You will recall that they found that donating blood four times per year lowered systolic blood pressures an average of 12 points, presumably through improvements in the Methuselah Factor.[91]

Now, on balance, not every scientist thinks that blood donation is of unqualified benefit. There is some evidence that donating blood as your *sole* Methuselah Factor boosting strategy is probably not optimal. If you are not making other positive lifestyle changes, regular blood donation may actually worsen some of your blood fats, lowering your good HDL and undesirably raising levels of a blood fat called triglycerides.[92] But don't worry. As you embark on the comprehensive lifestyle program outlined on these pages, you'll be following a plan calculated to help you reap the benefits of blood donation on your Methuselah Factor, *plus* improve your blood fats.

So, here's your challenge for today: Get on the phone and call your local blood bank. The purpose of the call is to find out where they are located and then make plans to donate blood. I'd like to encourage you to plan that blood donation during this thirty-day program. Sooner is better.

Already a blood donor? Check and see if it is too soon to donate again. You've been turned down as a donor before? Call anyway. The criteria for blood donors change over time. Your body changes as well. Someone who wasn't qualified to donate blood last year may be a candidate today.

For some of you this is a tough challenge. The very thought of blood and needles makes you squeamish. However, I'm *not* asking you to *donate blood*. I'm just asking you to *make a call*. But, yes, I did encourage you to be bold, so that might mean you'll actually part with some of your blood.

For others of you, especially if you've donated blood before and realize how safe and generally painless the process is, today's task might seem too easy. But don't worry, I'll be raising the bar shortly.

Before we end, revisit Figure 15. As I explained in the previous chapter, if you've already called the blood bank, put an "X" in the box for the row corresponding to Day 1 in the column listing today's task, "Call a local blood bank." When tomorrow comes, you can drop down to the next row, and again put an "X" in the box. Again, unlike the rest of my daily challenges, this assignment you must complete only once during the program. However, don't fill an "X" in every box in the "Call a local blood bank" column in advance. Even if you called the blood bank at the beginning of the program, I still want you to wait until the day in question before filling in any given box. Why? Because I want you at least to be *thinking* about blood donation every day this month. After all, I'm hoping that many of you will do more than just *call* the blood bank. You'll get the most benefit if you actually *donate* blood this month. And the sooner you do it, the better.

16

DAY 2: MEASURE, MEASURE, MEASURE

Today's Challenge: Make a commitment to track at least one measurement throughout the course of this program (e.g., blood pressure, blood sugar, weight, etc.).

YEARS AGO, TWO WOMEN attended a residential medical program where I worked. They had both traveled hundreds of miles with hopes of getting their diabetes under control. Early in the program, one of the things we asked them was today's challenge: to *measure, measure, measure*—in this case, their blood sugars.

Blood sugar measurement has never been the most enjoyable of medical activities. True, the lancets (those little pricking devices that cause you to bleed) have gotten smaller and smaller over the years. Nonetheless, they still can cause some discomfort or pain. Consequently, these ladies were not enamored at the thought of frequent blood sugar testing. (We asked them to check their sugars before, and then two hours after, each meal.) However, they complied.

Both women quickly realized the power of measurement. Being aware of their blood sugars allowed them to tailor their dietary choices to keep their blood sugars more stable. Some weeks after attending the program, they confided to a close friend that one of the keys to ultimately getting off their diabetes medications was careful attention to their blood sugars.

How could measurement help someone get the upper hand when it comes to diabetes? By checking your blood sugar before and then two hours after meals, you can determine what are your best meal choices to keep your sugars under control. So long as they're not getting into problems with low blood sugars (hypoglycemia) later in the day, I generally encourage my diabetic patients to try to keep their blood sugar from rising no more than 60 points within two hours of eating, with an actual reading at or below 160 mg/dl.

If you have diabetes and are a bit bewildered about how to improve your blood sugar, I have good news. The principles that help blood fluidity often help diabetes. For example, we'll learn that eating more beans can improve your hemorheology (coming up on Day 4). If you want additional practical guidelines on diabetes food choices, check out my free handout at: www.compass-health.net/diabetes-food-handout.

If you have diabetes or other problems with blood sugar, the message of this chapter is likely already resonating with you. As we have observed earlier, diabetes itself worsens your Methuselah Factor.[93] Therefore, addressing blood sugar abnormalities is of prime importance on your journey to better blood fluidity. Frequent blood sugar testing can be one of the keys to your achieving better glucose control and more optimal hemorheology.

However, many of you don't have diabetes. Are you then off the hook? No. I want each of you to measure *something* during this thirty-day journey. If you read my book, *Thirty Days to Natural Blood Pressure Control*, you know that I and my co-authors argued for checking your blood pressure three times daily while on that aggressive thirty-day program. And, yes, high blood pressure also adversely impacts your hemorheology. So, if you have high blood pressure, I'm asking you to check your blood pressure at least daily over the next 29 days.

Whether it's diabetes or high blood pressure, those measurements have another very important purpose. As your numbers improve, it may be time to have your health care provider begin to decrease your medications. At this juncture I should mention something very important: if you are on *any* prescription medication, but especially if you are on one or more drugs for diabetes, high blood pressure, cancer, heart disease or a transplanted organ, then you need to be in touch with your health care provider. If you have not communicated with your doctor, please do so within the next two days. Yes, I realize it's not likely you can get an appointment that quickly. However, at least check in with the medical office and let them know you're planning to make some lifestyle changes. Ask someone to let you know if there are special cautions. Let them know that you'll be checking your readings as you go through the program, and you'll inform them if your numbers are getting too low.

How Low is Too Low?

When it comes to blood sugar, if you are on diabetes medication and on a systematic program like *The Methuselah Factor Diet and Lifestyle Program*, I begin to get concerned when I see fasting blood sugars consistently running below 100. Remember, we're expecting blood sugars to continue to drop during the thirty days, so blood sugars in the 90s, which might be otherwise exemplary, may be harbingers of dangerous hypoglycemia tomorrow, or next week. So, in my book, blood sugars below 100 are a sign to start decreasing medications.

In the arena of high blood pressure, if the systolic (or upper) number is running consistently below 130, this is generally time when I begin decreasing blood pressure medications. (The lower number in the BP reading, called the *diastolic* number, typically doesn't cause problems if it is low in isolation.)

Now, when it comes to decreasing medications, at least initially, the emphasis is on *decreasing*, not eliminating. There can be danger in stopping certain drugs too quickly. Tapering is, usually, a far safer approach. For example, if one of my patients is on 20 mg of a medication called lisinopril, and their systolic blood pressure is now running consistently between 100 and 122, I likely will cut them down from 20 mg to 10 mg of lisinopril daily. If their numbers stay low or continue to fall, we may ultimately stop the medication all together. Nonetheless, that medication-elimination process may involve several stages, perhaps backing off to 5 mg daily and then even to 5 mg every other day. (Incidentally, every-other-day dosing of blood pressure or blood sugar medications are not typically a good strategy for controlling one's numbers, although it may be a reasonable way to transition off a medication.) Although I've provided some insights into how at least one physician's mind (mine) works, the bottom line is this: medication adjustments should be made only by your health care provider.

What if I Don't Have Blood Pressure or Blood Sugar Problems?

You have neither high blood pressure nor diabetes. What then? Monitor something of relevance when it comes to your personal health goals. Perhaps you're wanting to trim down. Then check your weight once per week during our thirty-day journey.

(I generally don't recommend daily weight checks. Weight tends to fluctuate from day to day. "Weigh in" too frequently and you're more likely to get discouraged by those daily fluctuations rather than impressed by the progress you're making.)

This is a perfect time to reemphasize something I mentioned in Chapter 16: regardless of the short-term measurements you commit to, try to get some comprehensive measurements that you will repeat at the end of your thirty-day program. From my perspective, anything that you measure within the first seven days of the program will count for your initial values. Anything measured on Day 28 or later (up to seven days after you finish Day 30) counts for your concluding values. If you can't come up with any other commitment when it comes to today's goal of "measure, measure, measure" at least commit to having some initial measurements and final measurements. If you can get some fasting blood work done to check your "lipid panel," even better. (The lipid panel looks at critical blood fats including cholesterol and triglycerides. Many of the columns in Figure 16 reflect values obtained from a lipid panel.)

If you haven't picked up on it already, perhaps the most important reason to measure *something* is to give you some visible encouragement over the next four weeks. And if you just go with the option of before- and after-program measurements, the changes in your measurements will be exactly what you'll need when it comes to deciding if you really want anything to be different in your life after this thirty-day intensive.

17

DAY 3: MOVE MORE

Today's Challenge: Increase your amount of daily exercise.

MANY YEARS AGO, I learned that starting on a regular exercise program could entail a significant amount of discomfort. While living in Minnesota, I began making steps toward a lifetime of greater activity. For a novice, outdoor exercise might be tolerable during some seasons in the Northern Plains. However, by winter you'll likely subject your exercise commitment to considerable scrutiny.

It took me a couple of years to realize that the days I had the most compelling reasons *not* to exercise (too cold outside, too busy, etc.) were the days that I most needed to prioritize physical activity. One reason for this was behavioral: if you want to develop a strong habit, persistence during difficult times can really strengthen your resolve. But there's a second reason. At least in my experience, days that offered the most compelling reasons to skip exercise were typically the ones where I needed the stress-buffering effects of physical activity the most.

All this brings us back to our topic of hemorheology. As we'll see later in this book, stress is one factor that can dramatically worsen your blood fluidity—and exercise can be a powerful ally in defusing stress.

Stress discussions aside, exercise can improve your blood fluidity in and of itself. Rachel Adams and colleagues at the Cardiff School of Health Sciences, in Cardiff, United Kingdom, looked carefully at how physical activity impacted blood fluidity.[94] They found a compelling dose-response effect, meaning that the more a person exercised the better his hemorheology tended to be. Additionally, they observed, in line with my emphasis in this chapter, "increased levels of physical activity improve the flow properties of blood and thus reduce the risk of developing cardiovascular disease. Even small increases in activity result in some reduction in cardiovascular risk."

So what's my challenge today? Yes—increase your commitment to daily exercise. Let me tell you one of the most powerful ways to do this. Commit to doing something that you label as *exercise for exercise's sake* every day—even if your initial commitment is only for five minutes a day.

Here's what I mean by this. Don't give yourself credit for taking the stairs at work or mopping your floor. Yes, that *counts* as far as your daily activity, but I'm challenging you to do something more during these thirty days. I want you to say, "I'm going to do my daily exercise today," and go out and take a five-minute walk or spend a similar amount of time on that exercise bicycle, which you hauled down from the attic. Better yet, ramp your exercise time up to ten minutes a day, fifteen minutes a day, or more.

Another Way to Look at Exercise

When you wake up in the morning, it's a given that you'll be eating that day, isn't it? Sure, you can choose to fast, and to drink nothing but water. However, barring such a deliberate decision, another day means another day of eating.

Similarly, you can choose to stay awake all night, but in general, another day means you'll set aside time for sleeping. Simply put, eating and sleeping are givens; they form a part of your daily routine.

By the end of this thirty-day program, I want exercise to be just as much an integral part of your day as eating and sleeping. You'll likely spend far more time eating and sleeping, but exercise will equally be a non-negotiable part of your day.

Could Exercise Be Dangerous for Me?

Most individuals can, without any particular danger, gradually increase their activity. However, there are several groups of people who should check with their doctor before significantly increasing their activity. If any of the following apply to you, be sensible, and check in with your healthcare provider first:[95]

- 70 years of age or older
- Known heart condition, or on medication for your blood pressure or heart
- Chest pain with activity, or new onset (within the last 30 days) chest pain at rest
- Problems with dizziness or loss of consciousness
- Bone or joint problems that can worsen with activity
- Awareness of any other reason why activity might personally harm you

What If You Already Exercise Regularly?

If you're on a good exercise program, *but you don't do something daily*, why not add a five or ten-minute walk on the days that you

107

don't go to the health club or do your exercise of choice? In this chapter my appeal for daily *exercise* doesn't mean you should do rigorous training every single day. I recommend against that; in fact, you'll soon learn that I recommend a weekly day of rest. But on that "day off" I still recommend *some* physical activity.

If you're among the minority of readers who are already on a daily exercise program, why not try increasing *at least some* of your daily exercise sessions by five or ten minutes? Alternately, consider squeezing an extra exercise break into your schedule.

Since more activity can lead to further improvements in blood fluidity, it behooves all of us to do more in the exercise arena. Before starting the next chapter, go to Figure 15 and indicate your commitment to a specific amount of exercise per day. OK, if you can't wrap your mind around a *daily* exercise commitment, then indicate your plans for how much physical activity you will get *each week* of this month-long program.

18

DAY 4: BE BIG ON BEANS

Today's Challenge: Eat beans daily (advanced, but optional, challenge: eat some beans at every meal).

ADDRESSING INSULIN RESISTANCE IS one way to improve our hemorheology. We learned this in Chapter 9, where we observed the compelling medical research link between increased insulin resistance and poorer blood fluidity.

However, knowing about a relationship and doing something about it are two different things. What can we do to improve how insulin works in our bodies (often called insulin sensitivity) and, in so doing, enhance our blood fluidity? One of the answers lies no further away than your dinner plate—or, if you prefer, your breakfast plate.

Over the years I've seen some interesting reactions to a novel breakfast item: beans. For most people any connection between beans and breakfast is non-existent. However, the amazing power of beans to stabilize blood sugar has brought this lowly food center stage. While working with residential lifestyle change programs, I frequently found myself and my colleagues extolling the virtues of beans at every meal of the day.

My own appreciation for the bean family goes back many decades. Years ago, I was a young physician who was just getting my feet wet when it came to conducting serious reviews of the medial literature. I was looking for connections between diet and disease when I ran across an amazing study with a captivating title: *A High Carbohydrate Leguminous Fibre Diet Improves All Aspects of Diabetic Control*.[96] In plain English, the title was highlighting exactly what a team of researchers from the Diabetes Research Laboratories at the University of Oxford found: feeding individuals with diabetes a high carbohydrate diet that included naturally fiber-rich beans improved blood sugars both before and after meals. Cholesterol levels also significantly improved on this program.

In the more than three decades since that landmark study was published, an amazing body of research literature has testified to the remarkable properties of beans. When it comes to diabetes, researchers from New Delhi, India, summarized their work in a publication entitled: *Antidiabetic Potential of Commonly Consumed Legumes: A Review*.[97] A more extensive review of beans was performed by Silvia Esperanza Suárez-Martínez and colleagues at the University of Querétaro in Mexico.[98] This research team looked at the far-reaching effects of beans to decrease the risk of diabetes, high blood pressure, cardiovascular disease, cancer and more. Of particular interest in current nutritional discussions, among the documented health-giving constituents of beans are phytic acid (phytates), α-amylase inhibitors, glycosidase inhibitors, protease inhibitors, flavonoids including anthocyanins, soluble and insoluble fibers, and lectins. This is not merely an academic exercise; some fad diets have tried to villainize certain of these beneficial constituents.

110

Take, for example, lectins, which have found themselves in the crosshairs of one popular diet system. However, as Suárez-Martínez and colleagues point out, these compounds have documented benefits in curbing appetite and in helping with conditions as diverse as obesity and cancer.

Sure, leaving beans out of one's diet might help a minority of people, particularly those who have an allergy to certain bean constituents—or for some other reason simply cannot eat them. If you're such a person, of course, I'll absolve you from today's commitment. But beware, don't eliminate all beans from your diet just because *some* have caused you bloating or indigestion. Not all beans have equal tendencies to generate intestinal gas. Furthermore, *properly* cooking beans from scratch can decrease the likelihood of digestive upset. Time-honored cooking tips reported to improve digestibility are the following:

- soaking dried beans in water overnight; pouring off that water; then cooking the beans the following day with fresh water

- cooking beans very thoroughly, so that they tend to fall apart with gentle pressure

- freezing your beans after cooking, then re-thawing before eating

Finally, we're not left to merely suppose that beans are improving blood fluidity because of their connection to things like better insulin functioning. Bean constituents like the previously cited anthocyanins have been shown to directly improve hemorheology by making platelets less prone to activation and clumping. This may partly explain the favorable Methuselah Factor effects on platelets documented by other researchers who studied various legume preparations.[99,100]

The case seems solid: unless you absolutely cannot eat beans, they are one important ally in enjoying better blood fluidity. For the remainder of this thirty-day journey, commit to eating beans daily. And if you want to increase your benefits when it comes to weight loss, diabetes control, and more, consider eating beans at every meal.

19

DAY 5: CONNECT

Today's Challenge: Connect with someone else in a way that relates to this program. (Electronic connections are okay, but face-to-face connections are preferred.)

A MEDICAL DOCTOR, "RICHARD," had become very excited about our book, *Thirty Days to Natural Blood Pressure Control.* His actions testified that his enthusiasm was genuine: he purchased three boxes (60 copies) of our book for his patients. So, I was not surprised when Richard wanted to talk with me about the book several months later. What I wasn't prepared for was the dialogue that followed.

Richard explained that he hadn't given away a single copy of our book. When I asked why, his answer was simple: "I'm ashamed. My own blood pressure is still too high." As we talked about the principles in our book, it was clear Richard wasn't following some of our recommendations. In other words, he could still do a lot to lower his blood pressure naturally. However, when it was my turn to share some advice, I didn't focus on any single neglected practice. Instead, I recommended a different strategy: "Richard, you've got to give those books out and offer a class in your office."

I wasn't asking anything onerous of a fellow physician. He had the books already. Our CompassHealth website also explains how anyone can complement the book with some inexpensive DVD resources and offer a seminar in their workplace, their home, their church, or some other community venue. (See www.compass-health.net/hypertension/.)

My advice to Richard was based on an important principle: When it comes to lifestyle change, the power of social support is real. In fact, when we focus on our current program, *The Methuselah Factor Diet and Lifestyle Program*, you're much more likely to embrace, and adhere to, my daily challenges if you go through this program with someone else rather than *going it alone*.

However, today's challenge, to *connect with someone else in a way that relates to this program* is not based solely on motivational grounds. It is also founded on scientific evidence. Social support has been connected with better blood fluidity. Consider one example of this research from Switzerland. There, researchers from the University of Zurich looked for associations between social support and poorer blood fluidity.[101] Specifically, in their study of sixty-three men, none of whom were on medications, the research team found that lower social support was associated with higher levels of the clotting factor, fibrinogen. Furthermore, when the men were stressed, those who had lower social support had greater increases in their already higher fibrinogen levels.

Okay, the evidence supports a connection between poor hemorheology and fewer social connections. However, you might be wondering: What exactly am I asking you to do today—and for each of the remaining days in this program? I'm asking you, on a daily basis, to connect with at least one other person on a topic that relates to our one-month journey. For example, you might tell someone at work what you learned about beans yesterday. Don't stop there; ask them if they have a favorite bean recipe. Or consider an example that relates to Day 3 of our program: ask a neighbor if he or she will be your walking partner for the next four weeks.

Realize, too, when you connect with other people you are not just helping yourself, *you are helping them as well*. Are you starting to catch the vision? Are you motivated to make a difference in your community? Believe me, this is not just author hype. Listen to an Amazon reviewer who used our resources on high blood pressure to reach out to his neighbors:

> "This is one of the best books that I have ever read to help transform my lifestyle. Although I was previously following several of the suggestions in the book, I decided to use this as a community outreach program in our city. We had dozens of individuals attend and I said that I would go through the 30 day program with them. I figured, 30 days isn't that long to try something. The truth is, in that short amount of time we had several within our group seeing their blood pressure either normalize or drop to close to normal ranges. Some dropped 50 points and have been completely taken off of their blood pressure medications.
> "For myself, I am sleeping better and have seen my blood pressure normalize. This book is just an incredible resource. If you are suffering from high blood pressure I cannot express how useful this book will be to you or your community. It's completely worth it's [sic] money!"

As I did with my previous book, I haven't left you on your own in this regard. If you want to reach out to your community, and help yourself in the process, we have resources designed for you.

Go to our webpage, www.compasshealth.net/the-methuselah-factor, for full details on free online materials and inexpensive DVDs that can be used to complement this book in a group setting.

What if you live miles away from the very person with whom you most want to share this program? No problem. Make sure you both pick up a copy of this book, then each of you watch my free daily videos that complement the material you're reading. You'll find them at: www.compasshealth.net/diabetes-bp/. Although initially branded as "30 Days to Natural Diabetes and High Blood Pressure Control," the approximately five-minute daily videos walk you through the very same steps that you're reading about in this book. As you might expect, the only difference is I limit my comments in the videos to things relevant to diabetes and high blood pressure, while this book takes in the broader theme of hemorheology.

Social support will be one key to your success on this thirty-day journey. Make plans now to connect with others as you seek to improve your Methuselah Factor.

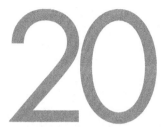

DAY 6: CUT THE CAFFEINE

Today's Challenge: Cut down on your use of caffeine. (Advanced, but optional, challenge: totally eliminate caffeine.)

IT'S NOT EXACTLY A rite of passage, but most Americans somewhere along the way rely on caffeine to help them push just a bit harder. Even if you're not a daily caffeine devotee, it's likely that during a crunch in your school days or an all-night road trip, you reached for a cup of coffee, a caffeinated soft drink, an energy beverage, or some other caffeine-laden option. For most of us, the caffeine helped keep us awake. But why?

Caffeine is a central nervous system stimulant; it also has the ability to ramp up stress hormone levels known as catecholamines. These properties underlie caffeine's well recognized role in promoting wakefulness.

However, when it comes to blood fluidity, it's also likely there are some other connections that you've not heard about. True, caffeine's diuretic (water-losing) effects have also been widely publicized. However, fluid losses from caffeinated beverages appear to occur primarily when individuals consume relatively large amounts of caffeine to which they are not accustomed. Habitual caffeine users seem to be protected from large diuretic effects.[102] However, any worsening of fluid status can worsen hemorheology. Thus, if we are truly interested in improving our Methuselah Factor, even mild effects on blood fluidity should not be dismissed.

Of even greater concern in the Methuselah Factor department are the results of caffeine interfering with a body chemical called adenosine. Current reviews, as well as older research, are consistent: one of caffeine's physiologic roles is to block adenosine receptors.[103,104] This may not communicate much until you realize that these receptors, found widely throughout the body, help to promote a healthy circulation by relaxing blood vessels, making platelets less sticky, and decreasing stress hormone levels. Consequently, when caffeine enters the picture, blood flow in our microcirculation suffers due to increased small vessel constriction, increased platelet stickiness, and elevated stress hormone levels.[105]

In spite of caffeine's rheologic shortcomings, most studies don't find evidence of significant increases in heart attacks or strokes when they attempt to look at these beverages in isolation. Think about it this way: no naturally occurring beverage contains *only* caffeine. For example, in the case of coffee, although caffeine may be undesirable for rheology, other compounds in coffee seem to have anti-inflammatory effects,[106] thus offsetting some of caffeine's dangers. This doesn't mean that coffee—or caffeine—is good for us. I would argue that instead of choosing something like coffee that contains some compounds that might be beneficial and others that seem detrimental, why not stick with options that are wholly good?

Let me illustrate this further. If caffeine and caffeine-related beverages were entirely healthful—and consistently improved our Methuselah Factor, we would expect to find that drinking more coffee would help us in all the ways that improved hemorheology does. However, even if some want to point to some encouraging data when it comes to coffee and cardiovascular disease, individuals who are slower at metabolizing caffeine (55% of those in a 2006 Canadian study), clearly appear to experience a greater risk of heart disease the more coffee they consume.[107] The researchers believed this increased risk was due to caffeine.

Just as caffeine may have differing effects on heart disease risk depending on the person consuming the beverages, so individual differences may affect coffee and/or caffeine's effects on cancer. Recent studies have linked increased coffee intake to increased risk of lung[108] and stomach cancers.[109] However, coffee might help prevent certain colon cancers[110] and skin cancers.[111]

All of this may seem to make the topic very confusing when most of us want to label things either as good or bad. My point is this: some things have more of a mixed effect, hurting us on some fronts while seeming to help us on others. In this thirty-day program, I'm trying to help you embrace things that will clearly benefit your hemorheology and increase your odds of living an abundant life. This is why I'm trying to encourage you to leave caffeine out of the equation.

But beware, the modicum of help someone might get from something like coffee may only be the result of how poor her hemorheology and other physiological characteristics are. In other words, if we really get serious about the *Methuselah Factor Diet and Lifestyle*, we may find that only the lifestyle factors that are wholly beneficial are the ones worth including in our daily regimen.

However, my concerns with caffeinated beverages far transcend the sometimes confusing literature on whether these drinks hurt or help our blood fluidity—and whether they hurt or help our health in general. The most important reason I've included caffeine in the first week of our program relates to caffeine's behavioral effects. As I'll soon demonstrate, even if caffeine itself had no direct effect on your blood fluidity, the more caffeine you use, the less benefit you may get out of this thirty-day program.

My concerns with the behavioral effects of caffeine date back some three decades, when I worked with the now late Bernell Baldwin, PhD—a genius neuroscientist who had a healthy respect for the behavioral effects of common drugs.

Baldwin told us that the great Russian scientist, Ivan Pavlov, had dubbed caffeine "bad-habit glue." To support the validity of Pavlov's moniker, Dr. Baldwin related how research on typists revealed that caffeine would generally help them type faster. But that speed came at a price: they made far more errors. However, the typists didn't merely make random errors; they tended to make the same mistakes they had made when learning to type. In other words, caffeine seemed to resurrect bad habit pathways that remained in the typists' brains.

I've tried to track down independent evidence of Pavlov's insights into caffeine, without success. However, over the years, I've found ample evidence of the connection between caffeine and unhealthy habits.

My most memorable personal experience came when I was helping run a residential stop smoking program. Patients would come to our facility for five to seven days while we helped them break free from nicotine. Because of insights like those of Dr. Baldwin's, we didn't allow any caffeine in our facility. In addition, we instructed participants to remain caffeine-free when they returned home.

We had the privilege of following up with many of our patients, weeks to months after they returned home. We were struck with an amazing observation: all those who remained caffeine-free stayed nicotine free. However, many of those who returned to coffee or other caffeinated beverages went back to smoking.[112]

Perhaps an even more amazing example of the connections between caffeine and bad habits came from a widely touted study published in *The New England Journal of Medicine*.[113] The publicized take on this large study (with data initially coming from over 600,000 people), was that coffee drinking helped people live longer. As one related press release expressed it, "Want To Live Longer? Drink Coffee."[114] But the data actually painted a very different picture. When the raw data was analyzed the researchers observed: "In age-adjusted analyses, coffee consumption was associated with increased mortality among both men and women." In other words, when comparing two people of the same age, the one who drinks the most coffee is most likely to die first.

However, here's where the plot thickens. Coffee drinking just happened to be associated with almost every bad habit that the researchers looked at. The more coffee someone drank the more likely he or she was to:

- Smoke cigarettes
- Drink more than three alcoholic beverages daily
- Eat more red meat
- Have lower educational attainments (complete less schooling)
- Neglect to engage in vigorous physical activity
- Consume fewer fruits and vegetables

Now remember, we've already seen that the relationships between coffee and health, whether relating to cancer or heart disease, sometimes appear confusing. With this in mind, understand that the researchers wanted to tease out relationships with coffee from other things that might confuse or confound those relationships. To do this they used advanced statistics called "multivariate adjustment for potential confounders" and came up with some very different conclusions. Specifically, when their mathematical models separated coffee drinking from all the bad habits that tended to go along with it, the researchers concluded that those who drank more coffee actually lived longer.

I don't think the researchers did anything wrong. They were asking honest questions and trying to come up with honest answers. However, their conclusions should be taken with a large dose of skepticism. After all, since the original data showed that coffee drinkers died sooner, the supposed benefits of coffee were not experienced in most of those consuming coffee—presumably because of coffee's behavioral effects.

Do you see that this article really makes a powerful case for what Dr. Baldwin said of caffeine years ago: it appears to be *bad habit glue*. Put simply, if you want to stick with unhealthy habits, caffeine (or, in this case, coffee) seems to be your friend.

On the other hand, if you want to get all the mileage you can from this thirty-day program, you would be well served by making a clean break with caffeine. If that's your decision, go to Figure 15's column for Chapter 20, Day 6. You'll then write a zero in the blank and circle the word *day*. In other words, your commitment will read: "Only have _0_ caffeineated drinks per day."

Does that seem like too much to ask? If you're not yet ready to completely jettison caffeine, then I challenge you to significantly decrease your intake—and list your commitment on Figure 15.

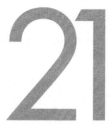

DAY 7: REST AND REFRESH

Today's Challenge: Make one day each week a "day of rest."

WORKING HARDER DOES NOT necessarily equate with working smarter. Abundant evidence testifies that overwork is deleterious to the human system. Athletes training for the Olympics realize that the success of their training is dependent not only on hard work but also on getting adequate rest.

Therefore, because it's my goal to help you accomplish the greatest benefits possible in thirty days, I want you to plan periods of rest in your program. Before too long, we'll talk about the importance of daily rest. However, in this chapter, I want to challenge you to focus on making time for *weekly* rest. That's right, as mentioned in my opening challenge, I want you to plan on taking one day off each week from your main day-to-day concerns.

If you're to really be bold when it comes to Day 7's challenge, you'll pick one day per week to walk away from all your work and school responsibilities. You'll lay aside as many of your life's mental stressors as possible, forgetting about your checking account, your investments, your aspirations for a better job, etc. Instead, you will focus on things like family time, inspirational activities, or time in nature, taking a total break from the things that occupy you on a daily basis.

For some of you, this immediately resonates. You come from a faith tradition where once a week your grandparents did just this. Maybe they called it the Sabbath or the Lord's Day. Possibly it was connected to the Muslim *jumu'ah* on Friday.

However, for those of you who come from a more secular background, such a weekly day of rest is distancing. You see it connected with religious traditions that have no basis in physiology. Don't let that stop you from seriously looking at my challenge. As we'll soon see, this concept of a true rest day seems to transcend spiritual considerations.

Granted, it may seem like a strange place to find secular connections between a day of rest and healthy physiology, but one powerful medical study suggesting benefit from the day-of-rest concept comes from Israel. Although that nation is steeped in a religious history that valued the seventh-day Sabbath, the authors looked at the practice from a secular vantage point. Jon and Ofra Anson of Ben Gurion University of the Negev analyzed a decades' worth of mortality data from Israel in an attempt to find any patterns.[115]

The Ansons discovered that death rates dropped significantly from sundown Friday to sundown Saturday, corresponding with the weekly Hebrew day of rest.[116] Their analysis suggested the benefit was not due to people merely having the day off. For example, other national holidays seemed to offer no mortality benefits. In addition, no decrease in Saturday death rates occurred among those who apparently attached no social or spiritual significance to the day, such as very young Jewish children or non-Jews who also had the day off.

What are possible explanations? One observation is that a weekly day of rest provides a powerful boost to social connectedness. A physician colleague once told me how, during his training, he was inspired by a secular Jewish faculty member who invited him to his home during his observance of "the Sabbath." This professor took time away from his medical pursuits to connect with his family, playing board games and doing other recreational activities. As we have already seen, boosting social connectedness in such a manner would be expected to improve hemorheology.

However, there is at least one other possible mechanism by which keeping a day of rest might improve our blood fluidity. It is this: the seven-day cycle is part of our built in biorhythms, and honoring those body rhythms helps to improve our Methuselah Factor. Years ago, the famous chronobiologist (time- and body-rhythm scientist), Franz Halberg, observed evidence in nature for life following seven-day (circaseptan) rhythms—even among organisms that could have no conscious awareness of our seven-day calendar cycle.[117] Other scientists, also without invoking any religious explanations, have seen seven-day rhythms as part of inherent cosmic rhythms. The Mikuleckys, father and son researchers, recently published data connecting the seven day week with a 6.75 day inherent cycle in nature that they connected to "the 4th harmonics of the Bartels solar rotation cycle."[118] Although other chronobiologists have recently argued that these solar rhythms are too weak to impact biological systems on earth, they agree with their predecessors: seven-day cycles are very real and are found abundantly throughout nature.[119]

Furthermore, medical science reveals that a disregard for body rhythms is linked to worsened hemorheology (which, in itself, demonstrates circaseptan variation[120]). One dramatic example is seen in rotating shift work, common in certain occupational settings where, over time, workers might be scheduled for various shifts that repeatedly disrupt the daily and weekly work cycle of the employees.[121] The evidence indicates that such irregular schedules worsen blood fluidity and its indicators, such as insulin resistance.[122] Those who do not honor body rhythms likely have significant Methuselah Factor impairments, as suggested by their experiencing significantly higher rates of cardiovascular disease that cannot be explained by poorer sleep or other lifestyle factors alone.[123,124,125]

The evidence appears clear: whether we look at biological rhythms or ways to foster more social connectedness in our increasingly disconnected world, we could all benefit from a day of rest once a week. Today's challenge is to make plans to include this in your weekly calendar, for at least the next thirty days.

As far as filling out Figure 15, I recommend checking the daily box in Chapter 21's column only when you actually keep a day of rest. Once you've done that, feel free to check the boxes for the following six days, since today's goal involves only a once-per-week commitment.

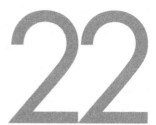

DAY 8: SEEK LOW SODIUM OPTIONS

Today's Challenge: Cut down on your consumption of salt (unless your health care provider recommends against this).

I'M NOT SURE WHO was more disturbed, my father or my mother. However, as a young boy I still remember my parents' mix of disgust and disbelief that one of our dinner guests poured salt over his food even before tasting it.

Although that might not seem like a common scenario today, most of us, nevertheless, have our salt consumption governed by habit rather than by dietary principles. The research is clear: we prefer to eat foods that are about as salty as the average foods we eat. I realize that this may sound like circular reasoning, but it's true. The person who eats a high salt diet will tend to desire far saltier foods than will someone accustomed to eating lower sodium choices.[126] (Note: many researchers talk about table salt and sodium consumption interchangeably because the main source of sodium in most human diets is sodium chloride, the chemical name for table salt.)

This brings us to an important point: you can start eating foods today that are substantially less salty than you now desire. Over the next several weeks and months you will develop an enjoyment for that lower sodium diet. In fact, as I mentioned earlier, research has demonstrated that an individual accustomed to eating a typical American diet can decrease her sodium preference by some 50%. However, it takes a full three months before the desire for lower sodium foods is fully established.[127]

So my message thus far is that each of us can likely decrease our consumption of salt, and enjoy our foods just as much—following a few months of patience. This, of course, begs the bigger question: why am I asking you to eat less salt for the remaining twenty-two days of our thirty-day program?

Sodium has long been associated with elevated blood pressure in susceptible subjects. (We reviewed this evidence in detail in our book, *Thirty Days to Natural Blood Pressure Control.*[128]) However, more recent studies are also linking higher sodium intake to adverse effects on inflammation and/or hemorheology even apart from its blood pressure effects. For example, researchers from Turkey looked at 86 patients with early stages of heart failure. They found that those who used more salt had significantly higher levels of inflammation in their bodies, based on measurements of a compound called C-reactive protein.[129] A larger study, also from Turkey, replicated these findings in 224 individuals with high blood pressure. Even if increased sodium intake did not raise blood pressure, it increased inflammation and the risk of high blood pressure complications like kidney damage.[130] Researchers from China were able to directly connect higher salt intake to hemorheology, demonstrating a connection between salt and elevations in Methuselah Factor determinants like fibrinogen and von Willebrand factor.[131] These changes could, obviously, be avoided by limiting salt intake. However, the investigators found that increased potassium ingestion could also reverse the changes.

One of the challenges with sodium intake is that it is affected by existing factors, like blood pressure and medication use. I've been encouraging you throughout this book to filter every daily challenge through the lens of your relationship with your personal health care provider. For example, if you are taking no medications, it is very likely that today's challenge will be beneficial for you. On the other hand, if you're taking medications for diabetes, high blood pressure, or heart failure, your relationships with sodium can be more challenging. Although many individuals with these conditions would benefit from reductions in their salt intake, it behooves you to check with your doctor before making any sudden changes.

How to Eat Less Salt

So, once you get the green light from your doctor to cut back on your sodium, how do you do it? Here are some tips:

1. Begin reading labels—and take action based on them. If a food has *more milligrams of sodium than calories per serving*, it is a relatively high sodium/high salt food. These items are best avoided.

2. Be prepared for some surprises. Right now, I'm looking at the label of a "healthy breakfast cereal." It has 100 calories per ¾ cup serving. Would you like to guess its sodium content? 180 mg. Yes. It qualifies for a relatively high sodium choice. (By the way, most breakfast cereals rate high in the sodium department, if not in the sugar department. With little or no sodium or added sugars, most varieties of shredded wheat are striking exceptions.)

129

3. Change your snack options. Yes, that's right; at this point in your program I've not asked you to make a break with snacks (although I may give you that opportunity later in the program). For right now, I just want you to pay attention to what you reach for between meals. If you want to keep things low in sodium, choose fresh fruits or vegetables rather than processed foods (those that typically come in bags, jars, or cans).

4. Watch your dessert choices. Again, many common dessert choices are high in sodium. Consider something like fresh fruit instead.

5. Eat out less frequently. According to food consumption data, the two leading sources of sodium in the U.S. diet are processed foods and restaurant fare. Eating out less frequently is one way to decrease your sodium intake. If you feel that you must eat out regularly during this thirty-day program, limit your restaurants to those that provide nutritional information—and opt for more low sodium options.

23

DAY 9: GET A GRIP

Today's Challenge: In addition to engaging in aerobic exercise, I would like you to add resistance exercise to your weekly routine (or increase the amount you do, if you're already doing resistance sessions).

I GOT INTERESTED IN preventive medicine during an era where aerobic exercise seemed to be king. Brisk walking, swimming, bicycling; we knew these were good for you. It seemed many of us professionals had our suspicions about weight lifting and other resistance exercises. Sure, those things might be good for building strength, but they didn't seem calculated to help your heart, your blood vessels, or (if we were even thinking about it) your hemorheology.

Perhaps my own gravitation to activities like running, ice skating, and cross-country skiing blinded me from researching the subject years ago. But now the evidence is incontrovertible, resistance exercises are good for our cardiovascular systems—and good for hemorheology.

In contrast to aerobic exercise with its rhythmic, sustained use of your arms and/or legs (thus increasing your breathing and heart rate), resistance exercise involves stressing your muscles against a resistive force. That force can be provided by things like weights, elastic bands, or specially-designed exercise machines.

Véronique Cornelissen and her colleagues analyzed the medical literature, looking for connections between resistance exercise and blood pressure. They identified twenty-eight trials comprising over 1000 individuals.[132] Their research revealed that resistance exercise had credible blood-pressure-lowering effects. However, I was most surprised by three studies that looked at what is called *isometric handgrip exercise*. The researchers found that particular activity had the potential to drop blood pressures in the range of 13 points systolic and 6 points diastolic.

If you're not familiar with the *isometric* terminology, it refers to muscular contraction without change in the muscle's length.[133] Imagine pushing against a 200-foot-tall giant sequoia tree. That tree is not going to move, so, no matter how hard you push, your arm muscles won't be changing in length. In the case of *isometric handgrip exercise*, a person holds a steady grip on a special device for a predetermined time. Here is one protocol based on research studies:[134,135]

- Perform handgrip exercise sessions three times per week

- During each exercise session, perform four sets of the exercise, two using your dominant hand, and two using the non-dominant hand

- Each set consists of holding a grip device continuously for two minutes at 30% of your *maximal voluntary contraction* (i.e., about 1/3 of the maximum force you could exert by squeezing)

- Take a one-minute rest between each set (therefore, the

thrice weekly sessions would each take about 11 minutes; four sets of exercise at two minutes each, plus three one-minute rests)

• Continue the exercise program for at least six weeks

Despite impressive published results, limited research has been performed on isometric handgrip exercise. However, there are already indications that part of the way it lowers blood pressure may be due to improvements in hemorheology. For example, some studies have found a decrease in oxidative stress associated with such handgrip regimens.[136] As we have already observed, such changes would be expected to improve one's Methuselah Factor.

Although the research is limited on handgrip exercise, a larger literature base exists relating to resistance exercise in general. Other types of resistance training do indeed decrease oxidative stress and improve hemorheology indicators.[137]

Yes, more research needs to be done. However, I believe that we have more than ample evidence to warrant including resistance exercise in *The Methuselah Factor Diet and Lifestyle* program. That's why your challenge today is to either add this form of exercise to your weekly program—or ramp up the amount of time you spend doing resistance training.

How Do I Add Resistance Exercise to My Lifestyle?

Of course, you could begin by adding isometric grip strength exercise. In fact, doing this alone would fully satisfy my challenge to you for this chapter. The only difficulty you might have is determining what constitutes 30% of your maximal contraction. A knowledgeable sporting goods store or health club should be able to assist you.

On the other hand, if you're looking for a more comprehensive resistance exercise program (which I endorse), the American

College of Sports Medicine (ACSM)[138] and other experts[139,140] have provided specific guidelines for starting or ramping up a resistance exercise program.

If you are already involved with weight lifting or some other program for muscular fitness, I'll assume that you either know what you're doing or have access to someone who does. Remember, today's challenge for those of you already on a resistance program is to consider stepping up your program—at least for the three weeks remaining on our thirty-day journey.

On the other hand, if you're new to resistance exercise, or have not done it for many years (and want to do something more than isometric handgrip exercise) I'll give you my synthesis of some recent guidelines in a moment. However, remember I already gave you some general cautions about exercise in Chapter 17 (Day 3). I am, therefore, launching into this discussion working under the assumption that both you and your doctor know of no reason the following activities would harm you. With that in mind, here are my recommendations for sedentary adults, drawn from current guidelines:

- Train each major muscle group once or twice per week using your choice of exercise and equipment. This should involve 8 or 10 different exercises. Note: "All resistance types (e.g. free-weights, resistance machines, bodyweight, etc.) show potential for increases in strength, with no significant difference between them, although resistance machines appear to pose a lower risk of injury."[141]

- Do two to four sets of each exercise with 10-15 repetitions per set.

- Use 60 to 70 percent of your maximum weight tolerated for each exercise. Alternately, start with a weight where you fatigue during the 10-15 repetition range (your *fatigue point* occurs when you can't perform even one more repetition with proper form).

- Wait at least 48 hours between resistance training sessions.
- For each specific exercise, once you can complete 17 repetitions at a given weight, increase the weight by 5 to 10 percent.

You now have the basics. Set your goals for resistance exercise. Indicate on Figure 15 whether your plans call for once or twice per week (if doing a general resistance program) or up to three times per week for an isometric handgrip regimen.

24

DAY 10: FOCUS ON FATS

Today's Challenge: Try to avoid saturated fat (generally found in animal products), and preferentially eat foods that naturally contain omega-3 and other polyunsaturated fats (generally found in plant products).

IF YOU HAVE DIABETES, and then took my counsel to heart on Day 2, you've been faithfully measuring your blood sugars. Armed with more personal information, you may have already stumbled onto one of the great paradoxes in diabetes nutrition: some foods that don't raise your blood sugar in the short term can predispose you to high blood sugar in the long run.

The foods most connected with this paradoxical effect are animal fats. That's right. Sit down and eat nothing but steak and bacon slathered with butter, and your blood sugar is not likely to rise. However, these carbohydrate-deficient animal products are far from your friends when it comes to optimal metabolism. They significantly increase insulin resistance, helping ensure worse blood sugars when you do ultimately eat carbohydrates.[142] If you think you can avoid the consequences of the high fat/high protein diet by simply avoiding the carbs for the rest of your life, that's not likely. Most people can't stick with a low carbohydrate diet for the long haul due to deterioration in mental outlook associated with lowered brain levels of serotonin and dopamine.[143] The bottom line is this: we all need to eat carbohydrates for optimal mental health. Do yourself a favor and stay away from the high animal fat foods and you'll handle those necessary carbs a whole lot better.

We've already learned that increasing insulin resistance is bad not only for your blood sugar but also for your blood fluidity. It is likely that this connection—as well as other metabolic changes—makes an animal-fat-rich diet a significant threat to optimal hemorheology. For example, researchers in South Africa looked at the habitual dietary practices of 1,854 apparently healthy African adult men and women who were at least 15 years old.[144] Better hemorheology (as reflected by lower fibrinogen levels) was documented among those ate less saturated fat (generally accomplished by eating fewer animal-derived products like meat, milk, eggs, and cheese).

In Europe, researchers with INSERM, the French National Institute of Health and Medical Research, published a fascinating study that involved another indicator of hemorheology, something called "endogenous thrombin potential" (ETP). A high ETP value is a reliable indicator of blood's tendency to clot, and thus an indicator of poor hemorheology. Not surprisingly, high ETP values have been associated with greater risks of both strokes and leg blood clots.[145]

The French team recruited 65 volunteers who adopted a lower fat, plant-rich diet for three months. Over the course of the study, subjects decreased their total fat consumption and increased the percentage of polyunsaturated fat consumed relative to saturated fat. (This occurred because their saturated fat intake dropped by approximately 50% while their polyunsaturated fat consumption stayed about the same.) With these dietary changes, ETP decreased by more than 20% on average, indicating significant improvement in the Methuselah Factor.

Among the specific dietary factors connected with ETP improvement was an increased intake of omega-3 fats. These fats help blood fluidity through a variety of mechanisms including decreasing blood viscosity, decreasing the number of red blood cells, and lowering levels of fibrinogen.[146,147] Although many people think of these fats as coming from fish (indeed, some fish are reliable sources), fish cannot make omega-3 fat.[148] Omega-3 fats in nature are made by plants and related species (like phytoplankton). Consequently, you can up your omega-3 intake by choosing more whole plant foods. Walnuts, flaxseeds and chia seeds are good sources of omega-3 fat.

There are additional benefits to avoiding animal fats. Not surprisingly, if you decrease your consumption of fat from animal sources, you're likely to be eating less meat. And meat eating appears to worsen your blood fluidity, even if saturated fat is removed from the equation.

One of these linkages between meat and poor hemorheology involves the mineral iron. Once sacrosanct in both medical and lay eyes alike, iron is no longer viewed as a mineral of unqualified benefit. Although iron is necessary for life, excessive amounts are linked to elevated hemoglobin and hematocrit, as well as increased oxidation in the body. Consequently, it is no surprise that higher whole-body iron levels (commonly reflected by a measurement called "serum ferritin") have been linked to a variety of cardiovascular conditions. These include heart attacks[149,150] as well as hypertensive disorders of pregnancy like preeclampsia.[151,152] There is also growing evidence that excess iron may play a role in dementia—and suggestions that regular blood donation, consequently, might decrease one's risk of Alzheimer's disease.[153] In one of the early studies that helped bring these connections to medical attention, researchers found that red meat and alcoholic beverages were the two strongest dietary determinants of elevated iron levels. All of these relationships are not surprising when we think about hemorheology. Higher iron levels generally translate into higher RBC counts and worsened blood fluidity. Excessive iron likely causes damage for other reasons, but its adverse impact on the Methuselah Factor still emerges as an important contributor.

The research is clear: animal fat (and red meat in general) is a loser when it comes to optimal blood fluidity. Therefore, one way to move in the direction of a healthier diet is by planning some *meatless days*. For example, if you commit to one or two days per week to go "meat free," you'll be on the path to significantly lower animal fat consumption. You're already trying to increase your intake of beans, so why not try a bean burger instead of a hamburger? Opt for a bean burrito instead of a ground beef one. Have an Asian dish that features tofu instead of pork.

Do you really want to up the ante? Then try a vegetarian diet for the remaining 2½ weeks of *The Methuselah Factor Diet and Lifestyle Program*. This may sound difficult, but a few weeks is not really that long—and you might be pleasantly surprised by your results.

25

DAY 11: SLEEP RIGHT

Today's Challenge: Commit to at least two sleep hygiene principles in order to help you get enough quality sleep each night.

IF YOU'RE READING THIS chapter on a work day, it's possible that you arrived at your job on time only because you set an alarm. Whether you were jarred to wakefulness by an old-school clock, or theoretically more gently awakened by a smart phone or other device that was monitoring your sleep depth, the result was similar: you woke up sooner than you would have without the alarm.

These ubiquitous devices bear testimony that most of us are cutting ourselves short on sleep. And the consequences of sleep deprivation are significant. For example, insufficient sleep is a dependable way to worsen your hemorheology. Harvard researcher Janet M. Mullington, PhD and colleagues elegantly summarized the data in their scientific review, *Sleep Loss and Inflammation*.[154] Among their findings: a night of sleeplessness or shortened sleep (e.g., four hours compared to eight hours) raised levels of several factors calculated to worsen blood flow. Among the blood components elevated by sleeplessness were: total white blood cell (WBC) count and inflammatory compounds like Interleukin-6 (IL-6), tumor necrosis factor-alpha (TNF-α), and C-reactive protein. All of these changes would be expected to undermine blood fluidity.

When we cut ourselves short on sleep, we also set into effect other metabolic processes that further compromise our Methuselah Factor. For example, sleep deprivation worsens insulin resistance,[155] a factor we have already learned was connected not only with type 2 diabetes but also with poorer blood fluidity.

There's another problem with sleep deprivation: if you can't function adequately the next day, you're much more likely to reach for that caffeinated beverage. We've already learned of the Methuselah Factor concerns with caffeine. Some of those concerns are the result of its tendency to boost stress hormone levels. However, remember caffeine is also "bad habit glue," making it difficult to break free from the lifestyle practices that have been undermining your hemorheology.

Think about it: lack of sleep is one of the key components in a vicious cycle that may well be keeping you away from optimizing your Methuselah Factor. What can you do? How can you sleep better and wake more refreshed? Is there hope for insomnia?

Each of these questions begs an answer. And the answers are largely found in the encouraging science of sleep hygiene. By following some simple principles, most of us can sleep better, and thus help our Methuselah Factor. When we wrote *Thirty Days to Natural Blood Pressure Control*, my coauthors and I summarized a host of key sleep hygiene principles.[156] For the whole chart, you can download a complimentary copy from www.compasshealth. net under the "Free Materials" section. However, to make that material of greatest utility for your *Methuselah Factor Diet and Lifestyle Program,* I've adapted the table into a check sheet that appears below. Your challenge in this chapter is to commit to daily implement at least two of the following practices for the remaining two-plus weeks of the program. Put a check mark beside each of the areas you select.

____ **Establish a Regular Bedtime.** Plan to get to bed at the same time each night, not deviating by more than 30 minutes, even on the weekends. Your body functions best when it can lock into a daily *circadian* rhythm.

____ **Get to Bed Early.** Because restorative hormones like growth hormone and melatonin peak earlier in the night, sleep before midnight is better than sleep after. Some experts recommend turning in by 10 PM.

____ **Have a Sleep Routine.** Your body does best if you give it cues to wind down. Prior to bed, consider taking a warm or tepid (lukewarm) bath or a hot shower. You might also consider listening to soothing music, praying/meditating, drinking herb tea, or reading something inspirational.

____ **Mentally Prepare for Sleep.** Wind down mentally before bedtime; don't take anger, worries or concerns with you into your bedroom. (Incidentally, watching the news is generally not an effective way to wind down.)

____ **Refocus Your Brain.** If you can't mentally unwind, go to sleep listening to something that is engaging but not stimulating. This is best accomplished by listening to something familiar. Such an activity can focus your brain on something other than stress-producing duties or deadlines.

____ **Exercise Regularly.** Exercise during the day but preferably more than four hours prior to bedtime. Exercise closer to bedtime can stimulate some individuals and, thus, make it more difficult for them to sleep.

___ **Get Bright Light Exposure During the Day.** Outdoor exercise during daylight hours can help meet this requirement. Bright light exposure early in the day helps you fall asleep; bright light exposure just prior to sunset can help you sleep through the night.

___ **Keep Evening Meals Light and at Least Four Hours Before Bedtime.** Although late night eating can make you feel sleepy, a rising blood sugar will undermine the production of growth hormone—a compound that even adults need to get peak rejuvenation from sleep.

___ **Avoid Caffeinated Beverages.** Caffeine after lunchtime may erode sleep quality. Even earlier in the day caffeine may affect sleep by lowering melatonin levels.

___ **Avoid Alcohol.** Late afternoon and early evening alcohol intake interferes with sleep architecture (the normal rhythmicity of sleep necessary for optimal restoration). Alcohol at other times can weaken resolve, making it easier to neglect to practice good lifestyle habits throughout the day.

___ **Avoid Nicotine Intake.** Nicotine is bad news for hemorheology and health in general. If you still haven't made a complete break, avoid this stimulant for at least four hours before bedtime.

___ **Ensure Restful Surroundings.** Cool, dark, comfortable and free of excessive noise are all qualities of an optimal sleeping environment. Wearing earplugs or blinders may be necessary in certain circumstances.

The rest of your thirty-day program begins right now. Plan tonight to put into practice the sleep hygiene principles you selected. If you don't see improvements within three days, why not add a few more of the principles to your daily routine?

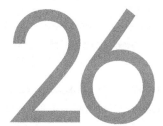

DAY 12: WATER UP

Today's Challenge: Optimize your water intake. Unless there are medical reasons not to, plan to drink a minimum of eight, 8-ounce glasses of water daily if you are an adult woman, or ten glasses daily if an adult man.

MOST OF US DON'T need a lot of additional evidence to convince us that nature's simplest beverage is also the best. If we didn't learn the importance of drinking enough water from a grade school health class, or at our mother's knee, then the lesson probably sank in on a very hot day.

However, one of the most impressive benefits of water drinking relates to something your parents or grandparents likely never told you about: hemorheology. In fact, drinking ample amounts of water may be one of the simplest ways to improve our blood fluidity.

Many lines of evidence testify to the Methuselah Factor benefits of drinking liberal amounts of water. For example, cutting yourself short on water has been shown to stiffen the membranes of your red blood cells and, thus, worsen your hemorheology.[157,158]

As expected by its impact on blood fluidity, water drinking has been linked to cardiovascular benefits. Consider the work of Dr. Jacqueline Chan and colleagues at Loma Linda University in California.[159] Chan and her colleagues studied over 20,000 adult men and women. Those who drank more water cut their risk of death from heart disease by approximately 50% over a mere six years. By "more" we're not talking about massive water intake. As little as three glasses of water per day separated the two groups, with those at highest risk habitually consuming less than two glasses of water daily and those at lowest risk drinking more than five glasses per day.

In Chan's research, drinking other beverages did not provide this benefit. In fact, those who drank the most fluid from non-water sources actually increased their risk of death from heart disease. This augmented risk *reached nearly 150%* in some segments of the population studied.

What About Alcoholic Beverages? Aren't They a Boon for Hemorheology and Heart Disease?

It's true, alcoholic beverages in moderation have been shown in *some* studies to help lower the risk of heart disease—*at least in some populations*. However, in other groups, alcohol consumption provides no heart or circulatory benefits. The best explanation for these different effects seems to relate to phytochemicals, health-giving compounds found abundantly in plant foods.

Since virtually all major alcoholic beverages are derived from plants, these beverages still have varying amounts of beneficial phytochemicals. Therefore, a person on a phytochemically-depleted diet (i.e., a person who does not eat many fresh fruits or vegetables) may get more heart benefit than harm from

146

an occasional glass of wine. However, when individuals eat a diet with plenty of plant foods, they get no added heart benefit from alcohol. This has been documented in the medical literature for over two decades, as testified to by the famous Oxford Vegetarian Study. When health-conscious vegetarians were evaluated as part of this study, drinking alcohol did not reduce their risk of heart disease death.[160]

Thus, if you're following the principles in *The Methuselah Factor Diet and Lifestyle Program*, you should have no need to use alcoholic beverages "for your heart." Beyond that, leaving off the alcohol should improve your blood fluidity—and increase your likelihood of good health in other ways as well. Consider the following:

- The U.S. Centers for Disease Control and Prevention estimate that as many as 88,000 Americans die each year from the use of alcohol.[161] These statistics are not due to just "alcoholics" and other problem drinkers. Social drinkers can also put themselves at increased risk of death. For example, "moderate" drinking puts you at higher risk of death from unintentional injuries like automobile accidents—even if you never become legally intoxicated.

- Even sporadic social alcohol use increases cancer risk, such that any alcohol consumption increases your risk of malignancy.[162] Among the cancers connected with beverage alcohol are head and neck cancers, colon cancer, and breast cancer in women.

- Alcoholic beverages have been linked to worsening a number of factors that impair blood fluidity:
  o Alcoholic beverages worsen insulin resistance, further contributing to derangements in the Methuselah Factor. This may especially be a problem in individuals with sleep disordered breathing, like sleep apnea.[163]

147

o Alcohol is a potent elevator of a blood fat called *tri-glycerides*[164]—and triglycerides worsen hemorheology.[165] The impact of alcohol on triglycerides varies with the amount consumed, as well as with lifestyle and genetic factors. However, if a person already has elevated triglycerides, a case can be made for total avoidance of alcohol.[166]

o We've seen how excess weight contributes to poor blood fluidity. (For example, recall Figure 9 in Chapter 9 that illustrated relationships between excess weight, insulin resistance, and inflammation). Alcohol contributes to weight problems in at least two ways:

- Alcohol is one of the most calorically-dense substances on the planet. Starches, sugars, and proteins all contain about 4 calories per gram. Alcohol "weighs in" at nearly double (approximately 7 calories per gram). Of our major caloric contributors, only fat (approximately 9 calories per gram) is more calorically dense than alcohol.

- In addition to packing a powerful caloric load, alcoholic beverages depress the frontal lobe of your brain, where wisdom, judgment, and foresight lie. Drink even a little bit and you're more likely to overeat—especially if you are someone who has to make efforts to curb your appetite.

• Alcohol intake contributes to bone loss (osteoporosis), high blood pressure, and digestive problems.

• Beverage alcohol interferes with the body's natural mechanisms to combat low sugar. Therefore, if you are prone to serious (typically medication-related) hypoglycemia, alcohol in your bloodstream could dramatically increase your risk of serious danger.

• Perhaps the most sobering thought (pun intended), when evaluated cumulatively, alcoholic beverages are major killers globally. In some of the most current worldwide data, alcohol is the seventh leading risk factor for deaths across the life span.[167] When looked at in terms of some of our most productive years, from the ages of 15-49, alcohol is *the* leading global risk factor for death among all genders, with as many as 1 in 8 male deaths linked to these popular beverages. Among the major life-shortening conditions linked to alcohol use: infectious diseases (like tuberculosis), road injuries, self-harm, and cancer. Is the solution drinking less? Well, that depends on how much less you are talking about. The researchers went on record, "The level of alcohol consumption that minimized harm across health outcomes was zero (95% UI 0.0-0.8) standard drinks per week." In other words, there is *no level of alcohol drinking that is safe when it comes to longevity.*[168]

Wondering about that "95% UI 0.0-0.8"? With any data analysis, regardless of how advanced the statistics, there is still some uncertainty as to whether what is being observed actually represents the truth. In this research paper this was expressed in terms of a UI or "uncertainty index." The authors were admitting there might be a small amount of alcohol you could drink weekly and not experience any increased risk of death. The *weekly* amount? Less than one beer (or, if you prefer, less than one glass of wine or one mixed drink—they all have about the same absolute amount of alcohol). That's right. The authors are saying that they are 95% confident (that's where the 95% comes into play) that, even if you could get away with no ill effects

149

from alcohol, you would have to limit your intake to no more than 0.8 drinks per week.

Don't chance it. If you're reading this book because you really want to have the best chances for longevity and high-quality living, leave alcoholic beverages out of your program.

How Much Water Should I Drink?

In Dr. Chan's work, the greatest heart protection occurred when someone drank at least five, 8-ounce glasses of water per day. Many experts feel that the five-glass level should be regarded as a bare minimum. For a better gauge of your water needs, some recommend taking half of your ideal weight in pounds and drinking that many ounces daily. For example, a 5 foot 4 inch woman who feels her ideal weight is 130 pounds would shoot for 65 ounces of water per day—or roughly eight 8-ounce glasses. There are some exceptions. If you have certain heart or kidney conditions, then your doctor may restrict your fluid intake. Honor those restrictions, as even moderate water intake can cause problems if you are already prone to fluid overload.

On the other hand, working in a hot environment robs your body of water. Even if you don't sweat much, heat can literally suck water from your body via the "insensible losses" associated with evaporation. If you have a question about your water intake when working in the heat, look at your urine. If you are well hydrated, your urine will typically be nearly clear in appearance. The darker your urine color, generally the poorer your hydration status. But be careful. If you have markedly increased water needs due to significant exertion in the heat, you may need to also replace electrolytes (blood minerals). For example, using an electrolyte drink like Gatorade® makes sense if you are running a marathon when the mercury has climbed to 98 degrees (37 Celsius). But for most of us, in most circumstances, pure water works fine.

One last detail: if you've heard drinking too much water can do you in, that's true. But if you are healthy and have a normal metabolism, and are not taking medications (like diuretics), the evidence suggests you would probably have to drink three gallons or more per day before you got into trouble. In other words, there's a large margin of safety for most people who set goals of drinking 5, 8, or even 10 glasses of water per day.

Now it's time to make a commitment to "watering up" for the rest of our thirty-day journey. Make a commitment to how many glasses of water you plan to drink daily. Indicate your decision in Figure 15, then chart your progress for the remainder of the program.

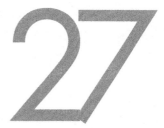

DAY 13: WATER OUT

Today's Challenge: Use hydrotherapy (water applied externally) at least weekly to address a specific health issue.

THEY WERE ONCE THE "poster children" for the pharmaceutical industry. Relatively powerful pain relievers, ideal for common orthopedic problems, a boon to headache sufferers, and safe enough to buy over the counter. Non-steroidal anti-inflammatory drugs (NSAIDs) seemed to have everything going for them.

Today the luster surrounding the NSAIDs has faded. This drug class has been linked to increased risk of a host of serious cardiovascular conditions: heart attack, stroke, heart failure, high blood pressure, and atrial fibrillation (a heart rhythm problem that can predispose to strokes).[169] Although once thought to have only blood-thinning properties, some studies now suggest these drugs have Methuselah-Factor-impairing effects. This includes increasing the risk of leg blood clots.[170] Either way, the message is clear: if you want to avoid the problems that accompany poor hemorheology, you'll want to avoid these drugs.

Wondering if you are already exposing yourself to NSAIDs? If you're using anything non-narcotic for pain or inflammation, then there's a good chance that you're taking one of these drugs. Because of the strong connection between NSAIDs and high blood pressure (research indicates these drugs can raise your blood pressure as much as 14 points),[171] we devoted significant space to this topic in *Thirty Days to Natural Blood Pressure Control.* We included an extensive table enumerating many of these drugs.[172] However, the list of commonly used NSAIDs (at least by patients in my practices over the years) is quite short:

- Ibuprofen (Advil®, Motrin®, Nuprin®)
- Naproxen (Naprosyn®, Naprelan®)
- Naproxen sodium (Aleve®, Anaprox®)
- Celecoxib (Celebrex®)
- Diclofenac (Arthrotec®, Cataflam®, Voltaren®)
- Meloxicam (Mobic®)

Few people in medical circles are arguing that these drugs should never be used. However, the longer the duration and frequency of use, the greater the risk of heart and other complications. Hence, the big question: is there a better way to deal with inflammation than by taking drugs with potentially serious side effects?

There is. And although there are natural supplements that seem to combat inflammation and, at the same time, improve blood fluidity, perhaps nothing is as simple and effective as the external use of water. (Don't worry. We'll look more at health-enhancing anti-inflammatory supplements on Day 27.)

Water as Therapy

Over the years, I've helped many patients with chronic pain. One surprising cause of severe pain, at least to the uninitiated, is diabetic neuropathy. In this condition, a person's nerves have been damaged due to diabetes' long-term effects. Although numbness and tingling are common symptoms, some contend with severe pain. I have had patients who complained of neuropathy pain so intense that they couldn't sleep or hold a job.

Like John. I worked with him when he joined me and my team for a 2½ week program at a residential lifestyle center. From the outset of John's stay, we employed a comprehensive lifestyle program, but we also used something called "contrast hydrotherapy."

Contrast treatments involve the alternating application of warm and cold water. We start with warm water for 3-5 minutes, and then switch to cool water for 30 to 60 seconds. To get a better mental picture, imagine John sitting on a swiveling chair, moving his legs from a hot whirlpool bath to a cool one at the specified intervals. A typical treatment consists of 4 to 5 of these warm to cold alternating cycles. When working with people who have neuropathy, we make sure to keep the warm water at or below 104 degrees Fahrenheit (40 degrees C). Because of impaired sensation, these individuals are at increased risk of being burned.

There are also situations where we must beware of excessive cold exposure. For example, extreme cold exposure may be harmful for individuals with severe high blood pressure, arterial blockage, or heart rhythm problems.

John made considerable progress and credited the contrast treatments with playing a significant role in his improvement. Was that a reasonable conclusion? It seemed so. John said when he skipped the treatments, his neuropathy worsened.

Hydrotherapy's History

The use of water for therapy is not a recent discovery. Indigenous peoples throughout the world have often resorted to the skillful use of water for a host of maladies. For example, we have evidence of hydrotherapy in the Americas before European contact.[173] The sweat lodge provides one of the most pervasive examples of the therapeutic use of water in this setting. Although sweat lodges in Indian Country today are often connected with spiritual healing practices, this was not always the case. Historically, *sweats* were seen by many First Nation peoples as valuable for their healing properties—regardless of whether or not they were coupled with overtly spiritual rites. Sometimes referred to by medical anthropologists as "sweat baths" or "vapor baths," these treatments were used by Native Americans with apparently good effects for conditions as diverse as agitation, arthritic problems, and digestive ailments.

Whether we are using moist heat or dry heat, heating treatments have been valued by many cultures and have been validated by modern medical science. For example, a growing body of research literature has examined modern applications for the ancient dry-heating process known as sauna.[174,175] Investigators have found that sauna may help a variety of factors that affect hemorheology by:

- Decreasing inflammation
- Enhancing the availability of the blood-vessel-relaxing compound known as nitric oxide
- Decreasing insulin resistance

Connecting the dots, you realize that the medical research on sauna is describing a practice calculated to improve your Methuselah Factor.

There are many other ways to skillfully use water. For example, ice can be particularly effective in the context of bone, joint, or muscle injury. In general, cold applications are best for recent injuries (especially within the last 48 hours when pain and swelling

156

are present). Heat often is more beneficial in cases of stiffness or spasm.

That's the foundation for Day 13. Your challenge is to reflect on painful conditions where you may be resorting to medications like NSAIDs or other prescription drugs. See if you can't use some of the hydrotherapy techniques that I've mentioned, or research others that are suited to a particular condition you may be facing. You don't really have any aches or pains? Then look into accessing a sauna or steam bath at a local health club. (Even if there are no medical reasons for them to *avoid* such whole-body heating treatments, I still generally recommend my patients keep their initial exposure very short, say five minutes, to make sure they suffer no adverse consequences from the heat.)

At least once a week over the next three weeks, harness the power of water externally to either directly enhance your blood fluidity, or minimize exposure to things that might be adversely impacting your Methuselah Factor.

28

DAY 14: SEEK SPIRITUALITY

Today's Challenge: On your weekly "day of rest," seek to connect with spiritual principles or values.

TODAY, WE'RE CONTINUING A cycle that we began seven days ago: taking one day off in seven for rest and refreshment. If you haven't picked up on it already, this circaseptan cycle is built into this thirty-day program. Therefore, since we've come to Day 14 (another multiple of seven), we're again focusing on this theme.

If you already have a certain day that is your "day of rest" and it's out of sync with this program, I would encourage you to take a few days off. Only resume this thirty-day journey when the days in this program that are multiples of seven coincide with your day of rest.

Having synced this program with your own weekly routine, we're now ready to examine today's challenge, "Seek Spirituality." Some of you may have thought that was implicit in my Day 7 challenge. However, remember, as far as this program is concerned, *your weekly day of rest does not have to be a religious day* (although it can be, if that is important to you).

Just as a day of rest often carries religious connotations, so does the term spirituality. Although I don't typically site Wikipedia as a reference, that resource nicely encapsulates the broader range of meanings that are common when experts today speak of spirituality. Specifically, Wikipedia identifies spirituality as relating to "the 'deepest values and meanings by which people live,' often in a context separate from organized religious institutions. Modern systems of spirituality may include a belief in a supernatural (beyond the known and observable) realm, personal growth, a quest for an ultimate or sacred meaning, religious experience, or an encounter with one's own 'inner dimension.'"[176]

So, my challenge for you today is to seek spirituality when you take a hiatus from your regular activities, every seventh day. At some point in that weekly day of rest, take time to focus on meaning and purpose in your life. This may not sound important, but I would suggest it is vital to your success in this program and to your life as a whole.

Tim Herrera recently wrote a fascinating article called "Why Your Brain Tricks You Into Doing Less Important Tasks."[177] There Herrera summarized recent brain science which indicates that most of us prioritize urgent, rapidly completable, tasks over more important tasks that take longer to accomplish. This is true, even if an urgent task is less pleasant than an important one. One of the author's solutions to this phenomenon relies on carefully scrutinizing our daily "to do" lists. Although Herrera did not directly advocate a weekly day of rest that included spiritual reflection, he did endorse this, in essence, when he recommended that his readers clarify what is important in their lives by prioritizing time for "looking inward," with a goal of sorting out what is really important, "truly core to who you are and what your ambitions are."

In short, time for spiritual reflection is vital to keep you on track with any goal-directed behavior, including this program. I'm recommending that during the next few weeks, you make a point of engaging in such reflection once per week.

However, spirituality is also important in its own right, helping you accomplish some of the same endpoints that an improved Methuselah Factor offers. In fact, the similarities suggest that seeking spirituality helps hemorheology in a variety of ways. (We'll look at some specific examples on Days 21 and 28 of our program.) For now, consider some ways that the medical research literature suggests you might benefit by prioritizing spirituality and/or being more religiously involved:[178]

- Improved quality of life
- Better adherence to health-promoting behaviors (like exercise and proper nutrition)
- Better physical and mental functioning
- Lower blood pressure and less cardiovascular disease
- Fewer hospitalizations
- Quicker resolution of grief
- A longer lifespan

So how do you fulfill today's challenge? You do something specific to address the spiritual dimension of your life. What you do is up to you. Sure, it may involve attending a traditional religious worship service. However, it may just as well involve a walk in the woods where you take time to reflect on your life priorities. Furthermore, you don't have to leave your home to seek spirituality. You can read a portion of a book that nurtures your spirit, or challenges you to look at your life priorities differently.

Go for it. Today and every seventh day, seek spirituality and see if it doesn't pay dividends as you work to improve your Methuselah Factor.

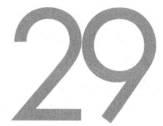

DAY 15: TRIM DOWN

Today's Challenge: If you are overweight, add another specific element to your daily program to help you trim down.

OVER THE YEARS, MY patients have thought it was one of the most difficult lifestyle prescriptions: make a clean break with one of their favorite foods. However, those who have tried it have often found it to be one of the most empowering principles they ever applied.

I think of Jane, a patient in a residential lifestyle change program. After one of my lectures, Jane approached me and made a confession: she was an ice-cream-aholic. However, she also communicated that something in my lecture resonated with her. During my presentation, I had spoken of the power of using clean breaks to make significant improvements in one's lifestyle. Jane decided at that moment she needed to take a different approach to dealing with her beloved ice cream. She told me she decided to leave it off altogether. No more "cutting back" or "just for special occasions."

Some months later, Jane told me that she had stuck with her commitment to ice-cream-free living. Having made a clean break, she was enjoying life, free of those cravings for "just a little bit" of ice cream.

I begin this chapter with an illustration of the power of clean breaks, because it may be just the principle you need to finally take charge of your weight. I'll share some other weight loss keys shortly. However, we need to remind ourselves of why this Day 15 challenge is important.

In Chapter 10, we found that poor hemorheology increases the likelihood that any of us will gain weight. However, we saw that the relationship worked in the other direction as well: if you are overweight your blood fluidity is, likely, suffering. I can't emphasize this connection enough. In a nation, and a world, where many of us struggle with our weight, our success in improving our blood fluidity may rest largely with our learning how to trim down.

The relationship between overweight and poor hemorheology is complex, but it appears to be related to a number of factors. First, fat cells, also known as adipocytes, are not merely quiescent fat storage chambers. These cells make inflammatory compounds.[179] Consequently, the more fat we store, the more inflammation we tend to have in our bodies. And the greater the inflammation, the worse our Methuselah Factor.[180]

Second, weight gain is associated with insulin resistance. Although some of this connection may be the result of increased inflammation, other factors may be operative as well.[181]

Third, being overweight is associated with other disturbances in rheologic factors. It can be hard to tell whether factors like inflammation and insulin resistance are responsible, or whether overweight itself causes these perturbations independently. For example, as one continues to gain weight, a number of changes

164

occur in his or her red blood cells that progressively worsen hemorheology.[182]

Regardless of the precise mechanisms, the case for a connection between being overweight and poor hemorheology is compelling. It argues eloquently for each of us to trim down if we are carrying extra pounds.

Over the course of thousands of patient encounters, I've learned that discussions about weight loss are often extremely frustrating to those carrying extra pounds. After all, most people who are significantly overweight would love to trim down. They just don't know *how* to have lasting success.

I've already been pointing to one of the secrets to weight loss throughout the pages of this book: improve your Methuselah Factor. Of course, that's what this entire thirty-day plan is centered on. However, some additional strategies can provide extra help when it comes to shedding some of those unwanted pounds. If you are overweight, today's challenge is to add, for the remainder of your thirty-day program, one more specific, daily element calculated to help you lose weight. You can choose anything, but here are some options:

- **Make clean breaks with problem foods and habits.** I've already illustrated this with Jane's case. The message is simple: if you have an addictive relationship with something, lasting success usually requires clean breaks, not merely cutting back. As professionals, we don't tell the alcoholic to just drink at special occasions. We encourage a clean break. Similarly, some of your most beloved habits may be addictions. Success comes when you leave those items out of your life completely. Identifying problem foods and eliminating them can be your key to success.

- **Increase your exercise.** I've already asked you to ramp up your exercise twice in the past two weeks. However, if you can't come up with another viable strategy, a decision to do even more exercise definitely answers today's challenge. In speaking about exercise, let me make a very important point. Even if getting more activity doesn't cause you to lose a single pound, the exercise itself will likely further improve your hemorheology.

Over fifteen years ago, a fascinating study was published by researchers at the Cooper Institute in Dallas, Texas.[183] The researchers were basically trying to answer the question: if you had only two options to choose between, should you opt for being "fit and fat" or "thin and unfit"? They concluded you're generally better off being overweight and in good shape than being trim but deconditioned.

For example, the Cooper team found that exercise alone could measurably improve fibrinogen, one determinant of our Methuselah Factor. "Obese" individuals with high fitness levels tended to have significantly lower (better) fibrinogen levels than thin folks who were unfit. Furthermore, if a person was very fit, losing more weight didn't seem to make much difference in the fibrinogen department. The message: even if ramping up your exercise doesn't help you lose weight, you're still likely improving your Methuselah Factor.

However, before you write off today's challenge to *Trim Down*, the Cooper Center researchers found that even if someone was "fit and fat" he could improve other aspects of hemorheology by losing a few more pounds. For example, white blood count, another determinant of blood fluidity, tended to improve (decrease) as participants lost weight.

Yes, exercise has benefits on blood fluidity beyond weight loss. However, if upping your exercise for the next couple of weeks can help you lose even a little bit more weight, your Methuselah Factor will be that much better.

- **Forget about your goal weight.** Years ago, I was the medical director for a large hospital system's weight loss program. I made a startling observation: one of the reasons for failure in the weight loss arena was unrealistic expectations. I would see patients lose 20, 30, 50 pounds or more, only to give up because they couldn't get their weight down as low as their sister's, or brother's, or husband's weight. Here's my point: I don't care what the weight charts say. Believe me: you're a whole lot better off at 250 pounds than 325 pounds. Trim down. Celebrate your success. And don't let yourself— or anyone else—convince you that you're not successful just because you haven't reached some "ideal weight."

If you don't have any weight to lose, my challenge to you today is to pay special attention to the second bullet point above. Continue to invest in better fitness if you want the best hemorheology. For the rest of you, you know today's challenge: make a more calculated effort to trim down.

30

DAY 16: BREATHE DEEPLY

Today's Challenge: Follow a daily program of deep breathing exercises.

PERHAPS YOU'VE BEEN EXPOSED to one of the most basic anger-management techniques: keep silent and take three slow, deep breaths. Maybe you've engaged in a common stress management exercise where you breathed slowly, and deliberately, particularly paying attention to your exhalation. As you slowly released your air, you concentrated on relaxing your muscles. Still others of you have attended yoga classes where your instructor had you focus on slow, deep inspirations and full exhalations.

There is no question: slow, deep breathing is a practice that for centuries has been purported to offer health-giving benefits. If such breathing techniques haven't been a part your cultural heritage or life experience, more than ancient wisdom connects us with these practices. In more recent history, the Russian scientist, Konstantin Pavlovich Buteyko promoted deep breathing for a host of maladies. Throughout many countries, "The Buteyko

Method" generated further clinical interest in the therapeutic use of deep breathing techniques.[184]

What Constitutes a Deep Breath? And How Slow is Slow?

Deep breathing is generally defined as breathing that significantly engages the diaphragm, the large muscle that separates your chest cavity from your abdominal cavity. If you are using your diaphragm properly while breathing, your abdomen will progressively protrude as you inhale; it will then move inward as you exhale.

Normal healthy adults typically breathe between 12 and 18 times per minute. When engaged in a slow breathing exercise, you will typically shoot for a rate around 6 times per minute.

Slow, deep breathing has been linked to a number of physiologic benefits. Many directly or indirectly impact the Methuselah Factor. Consider a partial listing of the benefits of slow diaphragmatic breathing.[185,186,187]

- Increased blood oxygenation

- Lowering of blood pressure

- Improved return of blood from the legs to the heart (a result of optimized blood flow through the inferior vena cava, one of the main conduits returning blood to the right side of the heart)

- Enhancement of something called "vagal power," which helps counteract stress-related stimulation of the heart and blood vessels

My challenge to you today is to add a new element to your daily program: deep breathing. Shoot for at least three sessions daily that each include at least two minutes of deep breathing. Why not plan to do one session shortly after arising in the morning and another when you crawl into bed at night? Squeeze another two minutes in during a mid-day break or your evening commute.

What We Breathe Also Makes a Difference

Air pollutants have been connected either with direct adverse effects on the Methuselah Factor, or with increased risk of circulatory disorders that suggest a hemorheology connection. Consider findings from a stroke and heart attack registry in central Japan. Investigators there linked increased levels of nitrogen dioxide (an indicator of increased traffic-related pollution) to a 60 percent increased risk of fatal strokes.[188]

Making the connection to hemorheology even tighter is emerging evidence linking air pollution with diabetes.[189] The diabetes linkage may be partially explained by pollution's role in increasing inflammation, and thus worsening insulin resistance, another one of our recurring culprits when it comes to impaired blood fluidity.

The connection between air pollution and diabetes is further illuminated by research on what is arguably the most pervasive and damaging air pollutant when it comes to human health, tobacco smoke. With over 7000 identified chemicals,[190] it doesn't take much imagination to surmise that at least some of those chemicals might adversely impact hemorheology—and diabetes. About a decade ago, Japanese research opened a fascinating window into these relationships: Tobacco smoke raises while blood cell count,[191] and as white blood cell count rises so does risk of the metabolic syndrome, a marker for insulin resistance.[192] This is but one example of how smoking adversely affects the Methuselah Factor.

The damage to hemorheology inflicted by smoking has been reported in the medical literature for decades. In addition to the effects on white blood count, cigarette smoking worsens other Methuselah-Factor-impairing components like viscosity, fibrinogen, red cell stiffness, and tendency of both platelets and white blood cells to clump.[193,194,195] Furthermore, even a single cigarette impairs blood fluidity.[196]

Consider another tobacco connection that may be due, at least in part, to Methuselah Factor impairment: dementia. Over a decade ago I was impressed with the brain toll exacted by smoking when I read the results of a synthesis (meta-analysis) of 19 prospective studies involving over 25,000 participants.[197] The researchers noted that *at the time of initial assessment* current smokers had a 79% increased risk of having Alzheimer's disease and a 78% increased risk of having vascular dementia. Furthermore, *when followed over time*, compared to those who never smoked, current smokers had an increased decline in cognitive abilities and a 70% increased risk of developing Alzheimer's disease. These associations were further strengthened by data from the UK's famous Whitehall II Study. They documented that smoking in middle age (average age 55) was associated with memory deficits and a decline in reasoning abilities.[198] Although this data doesn't prove that smoking's impact on hemorheology is to blame for the dementia connection, it surely raises the question, especially when we recall what we learned in Chapter 7 regarding the impact of the Methuselah Factor on brain health.

Indeed, years of scientific research have presented a convincing picture of the health- and hemorheology-impairing effects of tobacco smoke. In light of this, some tobacco researchers are concerned about the increasing number of Americans who are turning to marijuana smoking, somehow thinking that it is a safe, natural alternative. Surprising to many lay people is one expert verdict asserting that there is "chemical and physical similarity between marijuana and tobacco smoke."[199] And, clearly, when it comes to the Methuselah Factor and a lifestyle that supports it, emerging evidence suggests that marijuana is deleterious. Let's look at a couple of the connections.

First, marijuana, like caffeine, can undermine behavioral resolve, making it less likely that we will embrace healthier life-style changes and stick with them. Among the behavioral connections with marijuana are the following: decreased motivation, impaired decision making and complex reasoning, and decreased memory and attention span.[200, 201]

Second, marijuana smoke undermines vascular health directly. This fact has been documented even in animal models assessing *60-seconds worth of second hand* smoke exposure. Researchers at the University of California at San Francisco found that one critical aspect of endothelial function, known as flow mediated dilation, was impaired by even this small amount of marijuana smoke, just as it was with tobacco smoke—with one critical difference. The effects of cigarette smoking wore off relatively quickly, while the marijuana smoke effects persisted for at least ninety minutes.[202] Remember, the endothelium lines the inner surface of your blood vessels. If the endothelial cells are not functioning properly, circulation in your tiny blood vessels will be impacted. Such endothelial dysfunction is exactly what marijuana smoke causes.

And don't miss the significance of the fact that these changes occurred even with *second hand* marijuana smoke. When you look at the medical literature, it is really not surprising that marijuana smoking is harmful not only to the cannabis smoker. As with tobacco smoke, marijuana smoke releases chemicals into the environment, posing risks for "innocent bystanders."[203]

Help Breaking Free from Smoking

As part of today's focus on deep breathing to improve your Methuselah Factor, I would like to challenge you to make a break with all inhaled tobacco and marijuana products. And, yes, I consider nicotine a tobacco product. This, of course, also puts most vaping on the hit list.

However, I have some good news on the quitting front. Along with our theme of breathing, there is something that you can breathe that can actually help you get the victory over inhalant addictions. When running residential smoking cessation programs, many of my patients found the urge to smoke was dissipated by inhaling deeply of lavender oil. Upon arrival to our facility, we essentially traded them a vial of lavender oil for their cigarettes and smoking paraphernalia. But there was more to the benefits than merely substituting one inhalation behavior for another. There is a body of research demonstrating a stress-reducing effect from the use of lavender.[204,205] And with that stress reduction we would expect improvements in the Methuselah Factor as well as in commonly measured variables like blood pressure. In fact, that is exactly what we find with BP, as pointed out in our book, *Thirty Days to Natural Blood Pressure Control.*[206]

You have two more weeks of our thirty-day program to focus on breathing. Make deep breathing a part of your daily routine—and avoid breathing (even shallowly) of noxious fumes like those put off by tobacco and marijuana.

31

DAY 17: AVOID HIDDEN SUGAR

Today's Challenge: Make a concerted effort to avoid added sugars. (Recommendation: only eat refined foods with added sugar if they have at least five times as much "total carbohydrate" as "sugars.")

WHAT SINGLE DECISION HAS the greatest potential to help you shed unwanted pounds? Some experts would assert without hesitation: "avoid caloric beverages."

I've seen the power of such a decision in my medical practice. Patients who ditch the soft drinks in favor of water invariably make significant strides in the weight loss department. However, even if you don't have a pound to lose, sugar-sweetened beverages—and other foods with hidden sugar—must be on your hit list if you're serious about improving your Methuselah Factor.

Before looking at the science, let me provide you with a working definition. When I refer to "hidden sugar" I'm taking about sweeteners that don't announce their presence when you look at the food. Sure, we all know that most ice creams and cakes are loaded with sugar, but by my definition that sugar is still often hidden because, on most of those items, you don't actually see the sugar crystals or powdered sugar coating the dessert item.

The bottom line is that unless you are reading labels, you're likely consuming a considerable amount of hidden sugar and its cousins. Here's a partial listing of some of the items I'm asking you to shy away from for the rest of the program:

- Sugar
- Beet sugar
- Cane sugar
- Evaporated cane juice
- Corn syrup
- High fructose corn syrup

Why is Sugar Such a Problem?

Consuming more sugar (or its cousin, high fructose corn syrup) is one dependable way to raise your triglycerides[207] and, as we observed earlier when we talked about another triglyceride-booster (beverage alcohol), higher triglyceride levels impair hemorheology.[208] High fructose corn syrup wreaks further havoc by raising levels of uric acid, the chemical responsible for gout.[209] But there's more to the equation: uric acid further undermines blood fluidity.[210]

And, of course, as I've already pointed out, sugar is connected to another contributor to poor blood fluidity: excess weight. To illustrate, let's return to our opening observations about caloric beverages. Harvard researchers conducted a systematic review that looked at all the medical research literature dealing with sugar-sweetened beverages (SSBs). They concluded that "a greater consumption of SSBs is associated with weight gain and obesity."[211] The Harvard team asserted further that "the likely mechanism by which sugar-sweetened beverages may lead to weight gain is the low satiety of liquid carbohydrates and the resulting incomplete compensation of energy at subsequent meals." In other words, the calories you drink are not offset by eating less at the present or subsequent meals. For example, put away 200 calories in soft drinks after lunch, and you won't decrease you supper by 200 calories. Include a 150 calorie beverage with supper and you won't eat a meal with 150 fewer calories. This research team shared additional sobering statistics:

- Despite World Health Organization recommendations that added sugars provide no more than 10% of our calories, Americans get approximately 16% of their total calories from these added sugars.

- Non-diet soft drinks provide 47% of the added sugars in the American diet making them the single largest contributor.

- Sugar-sweetened beverage intake in the U.S. took off in the 1980s and '90s, soaring some 135% in those decades.

- At the time of their study, an average 12-oz can of soda packed 150 calories with 40–50 grams of sugar in the form of high-fructose corn syrup. This is the equivalent of 10 teaspoons of table sugar.

To illustrate the connection with weight and hemorheology, consider this: if you drink just one additional can of soda per day (without otherwise changing your caloric consumption or expenditures) you would pack on *an additional 15 pounds each year.*

The Candy Aisle in Disguise?

With this chapter ringing in your ears, I hope you will consider avoiding (or at least dramatically curtailing) your trips to the candy aisle. (Never mind that the candy often finds itself inches from your cart in the checkout line.) However, there is other territory in grocery stores that is a veritable mine field when it comes to hidden sugar. And that's the breakfast cereal aisle.

That's right. If you merely look at their nutritional information, you'll find that many of America's favorite breakfast cereals bear a striking resemblance to desserts. It is not uncommon for cereals—especially those targeting our children—to contain in the range of 50% of their calories from sugar.

Here's what I'm recommending when it comes to breakfast cereals, desserts, and other items with hidden sugar. Check out the Nutrition Facts label on any of these processed foods. It should look similar to the example shown in Figure 17. Scan down until you come to "Total Carbohydrate." In the example provided, there are 24 grams of total carbohydrate. Below this designation you will find a breakdown of the carbs into dietary fiber, sugars, and sometimes "other carbohydrates." In Figure 17, just the first two categories are listed; sugar accounts for 3 grams. Next you will take the grams of total carbohydrate and divide it by the grams of sugar. I am recommending that you only purchase the item if your division yields a 5 or greater. Such a score would meet my definition of a "low sugar" food. Look now at Figure 15, where you are keeping track of your goals and your progress. You will notice for today, Day 17, I have listed, "Avoid high-sugar foods." In other words, I'm recommending you avoid any food that gives you a score of less than 5 when you go through the process that I just explained, dividing the Total Carbohydrates by the Sugars. For example, if the Nutrition Facts label on a food you were considering looked like Figure 17, you would be in business. A result of 8 indicates a relatively low sugar item.

FIGURE 17 — Assessing Sugar Content Using a Nutrition Facts Label

NUTRITION FACTS

Serving Size: 1 oz (75g)
Servings Per Container: 2

Amount Per Serving

Calories 110	Calories from Fat 10

	% Daily Value *
Total Fat (1g)	2%
Saturated Fat (0g)	0%
Trans Fat (0g)	
Cholestrol (<5mg)	1%
Sodium (35mg)	1%
Total Carbohydrate (24g)	8%
Dietary Fiber (2g)	8%
Sugars (3g)	
Protein (2g)	

Total Carbohydrate
content of 24 grams

Divided by Sugar
content of 3 grams

Equals 8

My Encouraging Story

I hadn't lived all that long before I realized I had a problem: I couldn't go to bed at night without eating something loaded with sugar. One night it was ice cream; another cookies or cake. But the habit was ingrained. I wasn't calling it a day until I had my sugar fix.

It got to the point where I realized I had to make a clean break with what was one of my most treasured food constituents. The sugar had to go. I really made a clean break. Now remember, I'm not asking you to go this far today, on Day 17 of our program. But for myself personally I knew I had to make a clean break. No more added sugar, all day long, 24/7. If there was sugar or some similar concentrated sweetener on an ingredients list, I avoided the food. Even a low sugar cereal like Cheerios® or Corn Flakes bit the dust since that five-letter word appeared on the side panel: s-u-g-a-r. Sure, it was rough at first. But the amazing thing was it didn't take me all that long to develop an enjoyment for a new lifestyle. I began to have more relish for naturally sweet foods like fruits. I no longer missed those once-cherished desserts. And a few years later, when in an awkward social situation where I felt compelled to eat a bit of ice cream, the stuff actually was distasteful. Honestly. I'm telling you the truth. My tastes had changed.

That's the good news today. You can dramatically decrease your consumption of sugar—and enjoy your life just as much. You can improve your Methuselah Factor by avoiding sugar-laden foods and beverages and, after a bit of adjusting, still savor your meals.

32

DAY 18: EMBRACE A
HEALTHY ENVIRONMENT

*Today's Challenge: Implement one environmental strategy that
you will continue for the rest of the program. This step might
include decreasing the noise level of your sleeping environment
or getting outdoor exercise early in the day (if you have trouble
falling asleep) or late in the day (if you have trouble sleeping
through the night).*

IN FEBRUARY 2017 AMERICA'S tallest earthen dam captured
national and international headlines. Following days of unchar-
acteristically heavy rains, structural problems developed with the
main spillway for Northern California's Lake Oroville Dam.

Water flowing through the damaged spillway was slowed and
Lake Oroville quickly reached historic levels. Those rising waters
necessitated use of a never-before-needed emergency spillway.
However, this secondary spillway soon appeared to be on the brink
of failure. The specter of a 30-foot wall of water surging down

the Feather River prompted 180,000 emergency evacuations. Although this crisis was ultimately averted, other stories don't have such happy endings: the nuclear catastrophe at Chernobyl; oil spills from super tankers like the Exxon Valdez; the release of lethal chemicals in Bhopal, India. Environmental disasters can take a staggering toll on life and health in short order.

Such extreme environmental events grab headlines, mesmerize audiences, and sometimes claim scores of innocent lives. However, they occur far less frequently than common environmental threats, which may ultimately cost many more lives. One way that those threats rob us of life and health is through impairments in blood fluidity. Indeed, when it comes to optimizing our Methuselah Factor, there is no question that the environment clearly has a role.

For the last four years I've been working part-time in a rural health clinic. One of the perpetual challenges that we face is a lack of providers. Recently I was comparing notes with a couple of other doctors who also work in rural areas. Both said that staffing issues were challenges in their communities as well. "Most physicians don't like living in rural areas," one asserted. "They get habituated to life in the big city during med school and residency and want to continue to enjoy the amenities of urban living."

Whether or not that hypothesis is true, one thing is certain: Life in a major city promises many benefits that country living does not afford. However, when we look at environmental health, rural locations seem to have a lot going for them. In fact, if you want to optimize your Methuselah Factor, you could make a strong case for living in a less urban environment.

Noise and Hemorheology

When we speak about urban environments and pollution, few think about noise—even in the public health sector. But more and more research is pointing to the dangers of *noise pollution*.

Monica Hammer and colleagues from the University of Michigan reviewed documented mechanisms by which noise can undermine health—and a number of these directly impact hemorheology.[212] Two are especially worth noting:

Increased stress hormone levels. People may feel that they have gotten accustomed to the chronic noises around their residence, such as the jet engines of a nearby airport, the trains running on tracks through their neighborhood, or the nearby road traffic noise. After just a few weeks of relocating to such noisy environments, "None of those things bother me anymore," and "I just sleep right through it all" might seem like honest testimonies. However, Hammer and her colleagues observed: "People in noisy environments experience a subjective habituation to noise, but their cardiovascular system does not habituate and still experiences activations of the sympathetic nervous system... The body's initial startle response to noise is activation of the sympathetic (fight or flight) part of the nervous system, similar to the preparations the body makes just before waking in the morning."[213]

In other words, live in a noisy environment and your stress hormone system will be activated throughout the night. The results can be seen in worse hemorheologic parameters, higher blood pressures, and even heart disease.

Decreased sleep quality. There are convincing linkages between noise pollution and the erosion of high-quality sleep. This should now come as no surprise. After all, if your stress hormone system is being activated by ambient noises, it is not much of a stretch to realize that this might have a negative impact on your sleep quality. That toll on sleep feeds back into your stress system, adding to a vicious cycle. Listen to how the University of Michigan researchers encapsulated this: "Disordered sleep is associated with increased levels of stress hormones. Microarousals [subconscious awakenings] appear to be associated with increased lipids [like cholesterol] and cortisol levels [stress hormones], and feed into the same pathway of disordered sleep, even priming the neuroendocrine stress response in some individuals to be more at risk for disorders such as depression. Increased blood lipid[s], heart rate, blood pressure, and stress levels from noise lead to atherosclerosis, which is causally related to heart disease."[214]

At this point a few cynical readers might be wondering if I have a real estate license and am preparing to make a sales pitch for some property in Wyoming. Realistically, even if that were the case, there's no way I could expect you to relocate in the remaining two weeks of this thirty-day program. So what can we do if we live in a noisy environment?

Researchers have found that relatively simple things can make a big difference when it comes to noise exposure. Even if you can't move to another part of the state or country, you might be able to move *the location of your bedroom*. Moving to the side of your dwelling away from the busiest street can decrease the activation of your stress system and lower your blood pressure.[215]

Living in a one-room apartment? No problem. Invest in some inexpensive ear plugs. Wearing these at night can dramatically decrease the toll that noise takes on your body and your blood fluidity. Sounds too simple to be helpful? Even in some of the world's noisiest environments, like busy hospital wards, simple devices like ear plugs and eye shades can measurably improve sleep quality.[216]

Air Pollution

As far as the numbers affected and the magnitude of complications, the single worst air pollutant is cigarette smoke. In Chapter 30, we looked at some of the evidence linking smoking to poorer hemorheology. Among smoking's Methuselah-Factor-worsening changes were increases in white blood count, viscosity, fibrinogen, red cell stiffness, and platelet aggregation.

Other air pollutants also can undermine blood fluidity and further increase our risk of problems associated with a poor Methuselah Factor. For example, elevations in white blood cell counts and fibrinogen have been linked to exposure to air pollutants.[217, 218]

Just as medical evidence connects cigarette smoking and dementia, so does data support a connection between air pollution in general and cognitive decline, including Alzheimer's Disease.[219] When looked at separately, other characteristics of the urban environment, like noise, emerge alongside of air pollution as risk factors for dementia.[220] The research challenge is this: because noise pollution and air pollution typically occur side-by-side, are they each culprits when it comes to dementia risk, or is one or the other merely an innocent bystander? Current research indicates that both air pollution and noise pollution increase our risk for dementia.[221] Although multiple biologic factors are likely involved in these connections, some appear to involve blood circulation.[222] Such a linkage suggests that pollution-related impairment of the Methuselah Factor may be part of the explanation for dementia risk.

Ultimately, moving to a more rural location may be a reasonable component of your *long-term* strategy for improving your hemorheology. However, since most of you will not be able to move to a more pristine respiratory setting over the next two weeks, are there ways of limiting exposure other than wearing a high efficiency mask or respirator 24/7? For one, you can choose when and where you do your most vigorous physical activity. A health club with a good air filtration system might prove a better setting for a workout than jogging alongside a major road during rush hour. If you're like me and prefer outdoor exercise, choose lower traffic times of day to get out in the "fresh" air.

Sunshine and Vitamin D

Noise pollution and air pollution may seem largely out of our control, at least in the short term. However, generally within our reach is a third environmental element, judicious sunlight exposure.

Sun exposure is the main way that humans make Vitamin D, a powerful vitamin-hormone that has far reaching effects on bone health, the immune system and on hemorheology. With respect to the Methuselah Factor, research has connected vitamin D deficiency with worsened inflammation and poorer blood fluidity.[223]

I realize that we have been cautioned about injudicious sun exposure for many years. That messaging is important. However, in our rush for sunscreens and sun protective gear, many of us have lost sight of one of the sun's natural blood fluidity benefits—the gift of vitamin D. If you think this isn't an issue for you because you're outdoors a lot, don't be so sure. A physician friend of mine recently told me, "Any patient I see who is not taking a vitamin D supplement, I assume is vitamin D deficient until proven otherwise." He could make such a statement because of what many of us clinicians see far too frequently, very low levels of vitamin D, sometimes even in patients who appear well tanned.

The message is simple. Make it an environmental health strategy to get judicious sun exposure. For many people as little as fifteen minutes of sun exposure to their face, arms, and hands will be sufficient for vitamin D purposes. (Actually, the precise amount of sun exposure needed depends on skin type, time of day, and season. To account for all these factors, scientists talk about a minimal erythemal dose, the amount of sun exposure it takes to turn your skin a light pink. You need only ¼ to ½ this amount of exposure to your face, arms, and hands to generate enough vitamin D. This guideline even includes a buffer for cloudy or rainy days.[224])

However, beware. If you live far from the equator, you won't be able to get the solar ultraviolet B exposure to make the vitamin D you need. In Boston, Massachusetts this equates to four months per year where even liberal sunbathing will not result in vitamin D production. As you move closer to either pole, that figure can reach six months.[225]

Concerned about all the mental gymnastics that seem required to determine whether you're getting enough sunshine? Then have your 25-OH vitamin D level checked. Some preventive medicine specialists recommend shooting for a level of 40-60 ng/ml. If this doesn't sound like a good option, consider supplementing with 2000 IU of vitamin D daily. This amount usually offers a good margin of safety at the same time providing enough vitamin D to address even a level that is too low.

Are Snowbirds Healthier?

My wife and I marveled at Helga. Although she lived in the Northern Plains, it was not uncommon to see her in shorts even during the winter. We thought she must have an amazing constitution. That was until she had a heart attack in her early 40s.

It's now years later, and as I write about environmental factors, I have to wonder: was Helga's exposure to cold ambient temperatures, without proper clothing, a possible contributor to her heart attack? Now I'm not implying that her attire was the sole cause of that cardiac event (she apparently had a strong family history of heart problems), but there is some very interesting research coming out about environmental stress from cold temperatures and its effect on heart disease and Methuselah Factor determinants.

First, physicians have known for years of the connection between exposure to the cold and a greater likelihood of chest pain or heart attack in individuals with heart disease.[226] Research has suggested that some of the mechanisms may have to do with stress hormones causing blood flow impairments. As one illustration of this, researchers have performed what is called "the cold pressor test." Historically they exposed a single hand, or more recently both feet, to cold temperature in the form of ice water. The results include a surge in stress hormones like cortisol.[227] Second, newer data is revealing evidence of higher levels of inflammation when humans are exposed to colder temperatures.[228] These lines of evidence argue for ensuring that we dress warmly. It appears to be especially important to keep our extremities warm. The practical implications of this suggests that it is far better to wear a down coat than a down vest. Similarly, we perhaps should think of donning gloves, wool socks, or long johns before reaching for merely the winter coat.

On the other hand, wearing clothing that is too tight can undermine blood flow directly or indirectly. On multiple occasions, we've noted the connections between increased inflammation and poorer blood supply. In this context realize that gastrointestinal inflammation can be increased by tight clothing, particularly if it compresses the abdomen. This would include things like tight jeans, restrictive belts, and compression undergarments. The connection occurs because such articles can increase the pressure in the stomach, making it more likely that acid will travel from the stomach into the esophagus. In susceptible people this can lead to reflux esophagitis, an inflammatory condition of the esophagus or swallowing tube.[229] The necktie is another article of clothing that has recently come under scrutiny for its ability to impair blood flow.[230] These examples should suffice to make a simple point: dress warmly, but beware of constrictive garments.

Well, there you have it. Today's challenge is to implement a specific strategy that will decrease your exposure to air or noise pollution for the rest of our thirty-day program. If nothing else, start taking a vitamin D supplement or pick up a pair of ear plugs from your local sporting goods store or pharmacy. Not sold on either of those options? Then just commit to keeping your extremities well clothed when faced with cooler ambient temperatures.

33

DAY 19: GO GREEN

Today's Challenge: Eat more green vegetables daily; consider fasting one day per week eating only leaf, stem, and flower vegetables. (Note: if you have any medical conditions or are taking prescription drugs, I generally recommend checking with your healthcare provider before going on any kind of fast.)

AS A PHYSICIAN WITH a reputation for using natural non-drug therapies, I have had many interesting encounters with patients who seemed to take "natural medicine" a bit too far. Some of those individuals arrived in my medical office lugging bags of supplements.

Now, it is true that medical science has testified to the benefits of a host of natural compounds. However, taking any of them in shopping-cart doses is a likely prescription for disaster rather than for optimal health. We'll revisit this concept later in this book. By way of contrast, I have seen many patients improve their health at the same time they *decrease* their supplement bills, simply by making healthier dietary choices.

The reason for this is that many of the most promising biological agents can easily be obtained from our foods. By making better dietary choices we can gain the benefits of natural health-enhancing compounds without exposing ourselves to the risks of excess (as can occur when agents are extracted from their natural sources and concentrated in pill form).

Perhaps nowhere do we see this clearer than in the burgeoning science surrounding phytochemicals. If you're not familiar with the term, "phytochemical" literally means a "plant chemical." In one sense of the word, a vitamin, mineral or any other plant constituent could theoretically be given this designation. However, in scientific circles the term is generally reserved for beneficial food components originating from vegetarian sources—excluding essential vitamins and minerals. In other words, phytochemicals are natural plant compounds that are not essential for life yet can benefit human health in a variety of ways.

Many isolated phytochemicals have become bestsellers in drug stores, health food establishments and on-line sites. Some of these compounds are household names. Others are essentially unknown outside the research community. Figure 18 lists some examples of individual phytochemicals and phytochemical classes.

My goal in this chapter is not to give you a shopping list of supplements, but rather to encourage you to make more health-enhancing food choices. One of the best ways to do this is by simply eating more plant foods. Let me illustrate.

A Real-Life Case Study

My grandfather, Santo, lived into his 90s. In addition to his age, a number of lines of evidence suggest he had a reasonably good Methuselah Factor. One of those pieces of data relates to his consumption of phytochemicals.

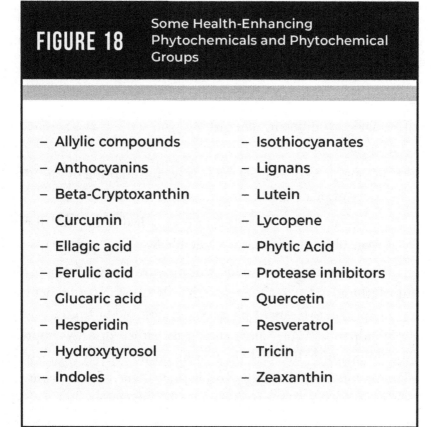

FIGURE 18 Some Health-Enhancing Phytochemicals and Phytochemical Groups

– Allylic compounds	– Isothiocyanates
– Anthocyanins	– Lignans
– Beta-Cryptoxanthin	– Lutein
– Curcumin	– Lycopene
– Ellagic acid	– Phytic Acid
– Ferulic acid	– Protease inhibitors
– Glucaric acid	– Quercetin
– Hesperidin	– Resveratrol
– Hydroxytyrosol	– Tricin
– Indoles	– Zeaxanthin

Now, I'm quite sure Grandpa Santo never took any phytochemical supplements. For example, I would be very surprised if he had even *heard* of anthocyanins, a particular class of phytochemicals demonstrated to have favorable hemorheologic effects.[231] Nonetheless, I know he consumed anthocyanins in liberal quantities.

Why? Because of his dietary practices. Grandpa Santo lived his first 21 years in Sicily—and continued many of the dietary practices he developed at a young age. Throughout his life he ate an abundance of green leafy vegetables, but also consumed liberal amounts of garlic, onions, tomatoes, and grapes—all rich sources of anthocyanins.

What's my point? If you eat lots of fruits and vegetables you *will* get an abundance of phytochemicals. In fact, you'll even be stocking up on phytochemicals that you have never heard of—and even many that have yet to be identified!

Stocking Up on Phytochemicals

For today's assignment, I'm asking you to do either one of two things:

- Commit to increasing your daily consumption of one category of plant foods: green leafy vegetables
- Fast one day per week eating only leaf, stem, and flower vegetables (I call this a "vegetable fast" in Figure 15)

Either of these two options will provide a powerful boost to your Methuselah Factor. The research is convincing that a diet rich in plant products tends to produce the best blood from a rheology standpoint. Many phytochemicals either directly improve blood fluidity or indirectly help your hemorheology by combatting inflammation or oxidation.[232] To illustrate some of these connections, consider the example of the platelet. Oxidation makes these clotting cells stickier and more likely to clump, characteristics that worsen blood fluidity.[233] Consequently, antioxidant phytochemicals keep your platelets more docile, leading to better hemorheology. Plants and plant constituents shown to help your platelets include:[234,235]

- Garlic (reductions in platelet aggregation of over 50%)
- Nitrate-rich plants (like green leafy vegetables)
- Resveratrol (from grapes)
- Quercetin (a ubiquitous phytochemical)

The Methuselah-Factor-benefits of eating more plant foods result from more than phytochemical constituents. As one

194

example, when compared to animal sources of nutrition, plant products have a superior fat composition in terms of blood fluidity effects. Better fats mean more flexible cell membranes. And when your red blood cell membranes are more flexible you experience improved blood fluidity.[236]

Putting Green Power to Work

Now the work begins. Conceptually, today's assignment is simple. I merely want you to make a commitment to either eating more green leafy vegetables daily or doing a modified vegetable fast once per week.

If you choose the former option, I want to challenge you to make a commitment to eating a *minimum* volume of raw green leafy vegetables *each day*. By volume, I mean something defined in term of cups; e.g., ½ cup, 1 cup, or 2 cups. What I'm looking for here, is your personal goal for the number of servings you'll eat. You can always choose to eat more. If you eat the greens *cooked* you get credit for double the amount of *raw* greens.[237] For example, a half cup of cooked kale counts as one cup of raw kale. Prefer to throw the greens in a smoothie? That works too. Just count the amount of raw greens you added to the mix. Doesn't sound palatable? At least try one of the options. And, remember, I'm asking you to do something only for the remainder of our thirty-day *Methuselah Factor Diet and Lifestyle Program.*

If even after your best effort, the daily greens consumption won't cut it, I've got another option for you. I call it the leaf-stem-and-flower fast. This special fast needs be done only once per week. This equates to twice over the remainder of our thirty-day program. During this fast you can eat any vegetable that is either a leaf, stem, or flower. This would include options like cabbage, cauliflower, broccoli, bok choy, kale, Brussels sprouts, lettuce, collards, asparagus, spinach, celery, and artichoke. It would *not* include root vegetables that grow underground (e.g., carrots, potatoes, beets) or vegetables with seeds in them (tomatoes, squash, cucumbers, etc.). You can eat the veggies raw or cooked. You can blend them in a soup or blend them up into a juice. (If you opt for the latter, you may want to hold your breath and chug that juice as quickly as possible. Most of the leaf, stem, and flower veggies have stronger tastes that don't translate into palatable juices.)

Of note, I have used the leaf-stem-and-flower fast for many years with my patients. It allows them to get the benefits of fasting on things like blood sugar and blood pressure without the magnitude of risk carried by total, water-only fasting. A total fast may worsen intestinal conditions like ulcers or gastritis. Total fasts also provide very little margin for error if a person has electrolyte (blood mineral) issues.

One of the interesting properties that make these particular vegetables good for individuals with high blood pressure or diabetes is their generally low glycemic index.[238] Glycemic index is a measure of a given food's tendency to raise blood sugar.[239] Whether or not you implement the leaf-stem-and-flower fast during this program, if you have diabetes, you may be interested in my one-page table that helps you make good food choices.[240]

Still trying to get off the hook when it comes to today's challenges? I will give you an out. Even if you're motivated to make the changes I'm recommending today, some of you shouldn't do it without first consulting with your personal physician. Let me explain...

Some Caveats

Eating more fruits and vegetables is a healthy practice for *most* people. There are some uncommon exceptions. For example, if you have kidney failure, compounds like potassium and magnesium can build up to dangerous levels in your body. Since these minerals are found in abundance in plant products, the red flag immediately goes up.

Certain medications may put you at risk from dramatic dietary changes. A case in point is provided by some high blood pressure medications which cause potassium retention. Those blood pressure medications generally come in two classes, ACE inhibitors (whose generic names end in *pril*) and angiotensin II receptor blockers, ARBs, (whose generic names end in *sartan*). Again, ramping up fruit and veggie intake may get you into trouble if you are taking such drugs.

Dosage of the commonly prescribed "blood thinner," warfarin (sold under the brand name, Coumadin®), has to be carefully adjusted when dietary changes are made. However, the old advice of not eating green leafy vegetables while on this drug is clearly passé.

Think about it this way. You're hospitalized with a blood clot, and fed that notoriously unhealthy hospital food. (Granted, recently many medical centers have made huge improvements in the dietary realm, but let's just play along with the stereotype.) Perhaps all you find palatable is the red meat, gelatin and ice cream. While eating such fare, your doctors put you on warfarin and regulate your dosage. Years ago, they would send you home and tell you to avoid a host of healthy foods, including nutritional powerhouses like kale, spinach, and collards.

Today, many physicians and dietitians realize a person can eat a healthy diet and take warfarin. The only issue is this (and it is *huge*): if you plan to make major dietary changes like the one I'm recommending today, then you *must* work with your doctor to regulate your warfarin dosage.

"Wait a minute," you say. If someone is already taking a "blood thinner" (whether warfarin, aspirin, or another drug) isn't their

Methuselah Factor already good enough? Not likely. Every drug bearing the moniker "blood thinner" works within relatively narrow confines—whereas *The Methuselah Factor Diet and Lifestyle* works more globally to improve blood fluidity. For example, aspirin acts primarily on platelets while warfarin's effects are limited to clotting factors associated with vitamin K.

The bottom line is this: if you have any question about the safety of these changes, or you are already on a medically prescribed diet, *do not change anything without consulting with your health care provider.* As we have noted, this would include individuals on certain high blood pressure medications, those with kidney failure, and those taking medications known to affect blood fluidity.

34

DAY 20: DEPEND ON YOUR DENTIST; MAXIMIZE MAGNESIUM

Today's Challenge: Make dental health a priority by getting regular dental exams and engaging in daily oral hygiene; increase your intake of magnesium (provided you neither have kidney problems nor use magnesium-raising medications).

IT IS RIGHT UP there with speaking in public. There is nothing most people would like to avoid more than the dentist. As a primary care physician, I have seen the results up close. Over the years, even cursory exams of patients' mouths often reveal an abundance of dental pathology.

We sometimes talk about how dental disease can affect your smile or your ability to eat certain foods. These are important considerations. But perhaps the most damaging effect of poor dental health is its impact on the Methuselah Factor.

Even if your teeth are fine, unhealthy gums can take a huge

toll on blood fluidity. Inflammation of the gums, known as *gingivitis*, has been linked to a number of factors that worsen blood fluidity, including:[241]

- Elevated plasma viscosity
- Greater tendency for red blood cells to clump (technically called *erythrocyte aggregation tendency*)
- Elevated fibrinogen levels

How Can I Tell if I Have Gingivitis?

Early on, gingivitis may not announce its presence. You may not have any oral symptoms and still have the condition. However, one indicator is a change in the color of your gums. Healthy gums are pink. When inflammation is present the gums typically become a darker, beefy red. As gingivitis worsens it can cause bleeding of the gums (often worse with toothbrushing), bad breath, painful chewing, sensitive teeth, receding gums, the formation of deep pockets between the gums and the teeth, loose teeth, and even loss of teeth.[242,243] The gums and related tissues are called the periodontium. Collectively inflammatory damage to these structures is called periodontitis. It is the main cause of tooth loss among adults.

The bottom line? Gingivitis and periodontitis are bad for your mouth, teeth, and blood fluidity. They are also extremely common. Recent data from the U.S. Centers for Disease Control and Prevention (CDC) indicates that 47.2% of adults 30 years of age and older have some type of periodontal disease, with that figure swelling to 70.1% of those 65 and older.[244] Remember, these conditions can do damage without a person being aware that she is affected. Therefore, regular dental checkups are important to both diagnose, treat, and prevent these conditions.

Because of the strong linkages between gum disease and poor

blood fluidity, an optimal Methuselah Factor requires prioritizing good oral health. Each of the following practices can help you improve your oral health, decrease your risk of gingivitis (or improve the condition if it already exists), and thus improve your hemorheology:[245,246]

- Brushing your teeth twice per day to remove plaque from tooth surfaces. (Plaque is a sticky film of bacteria that constantly accumulates on our teeth.)

- Flossing daily to remove plaque from between the teeth.

- Avoiding the practices of teeth grinding and/or clenching.

- Obtaining regular dental visits (generally once or twice per year) for teeth cleaning and evaluation.

- Ceasing the use of cigarettes and smokeless tobacco (Smoking increases the risk of periodontitis seven-fold.)

Today's challenge is to incorporate all of the above into your lifestyle. This may sound like a daunting challenge, but you should embrace it. Has it been over a year since seeing a dentist? Why not get on the phone and make an appointment today? That's a great place to start.

On the other hand, today's message may not be particularly challenging if you already have developed the good habit of regular dental care and checkups. That's why I have one additional challenge especially for those of you who already practice good oral hygiene: maximize magnesium. However, magnesium is so important when it comes to the Methuselah Factor that I want every reader to consider what follows—even if you've already been challenged mightily on the dental front.

Magnesium and the Methuselah Factor

In 2017 an amazing review was published by a pair of Slovakian scientists, Michal Pokusa and Alžbeta Kráľová Trančíková. Their research paper was entitled, "The Central Role of Biometals Maintains Oxidative Balance in the Context of Metabolic and Neurodegenerative Disorders."[247] Among other things, the authors tackled the far-reaching implications of lower than optimal magnesium levels in humans and animals. They found a number of connections between less than optimal magnesium status and poor hemorheology. Consider a portion of their findings.

In human and/or animal studies low magnesium levels have been linked to:

- Higher levels of insulin resistance and elevated blood sugars

- Evidence of greater oxidative stress and inflammation among those who are insulin resistant or overweight

- Worsened blood sugars and blood fats (triglycerides) in pregnant women with gestational diabetes

- Poorer antioxidant defenses

- Impairment of a calcium-magnesium "intracellular pump" in the immune cells found in body fat (technically known as *white adipose tissue*) [Poor functioning of this pump allows calcium to build up in immune cells, which in turn leads to their activation in the absence of a biological need. The resultant hyperactivation results in the secretion of chemical messengers (cytokines like interleukins and tumor necrosis factor alpha) which worsen inflammation throughout the body.]

By now, you realize that the triad of worsened insulin resistance, greater oxidation and heightened inflammation spells trouble for the Methuselah Factor. Consequently, it should come as no surprise that the medical research literature links poorer magnesium status directly to worsened hemorheology. For example, magnesium helps to decrease activity of the Methuselah-Factor-undermining von Willebrand Factor and makes platelets less likely to clump together.[248]

Other amazing connections between magnesium and the Methuselah Factor relate to kidney health and hearing protection. These examples further illustrate how the far-reaching effects of hemorheology exceed the benefits touted in the opening thirteen chapters of this book. In the case of our kidneys, recent data links poorer magnesium intake with a more rapid decline in function. The authors suggest these decrements may be due in part to the connection between lower magnesium levels and poorer blood fluidity.[249]

Magnesium, the Methuselah Factor, and Hearing Loss

For years researchers have connected magnesium deficiency with worsened blood fluidity and hearing problems. As an example, consider a 2000 publication that looked at the risk of hearing loss in an animal model of magnesium deficiency.[250] The authors found evidence that better magnesium status improved blood fluidity and decreased the risk of hearing loss under vascular stress. More recently, a 2014 paper found that US adults, aged 20 to 69, who regularly ingested more magnesium had less risk of hearing problems.[251]

Clearly, if your goal is optimal blood fluidity and optimal health, then you will want to ensure you are maximizing your body's magnesium status.

How to Maximize Magnesium

In addition to a critical role in hemorheology, magnesium has a vital place in maintaining normal blood pressure. Consequently, when I teamed up with Dr. Greg Steinke and Nurse Practitioner Trudie Li to write *Thirty Days to Natural Blood Pressure Control*, we gave magnesium a prominent place.

Let me summarize the detailed material in that volume in order to give you the two keys to optimizing your body's magnesium levels: 1. Eat more plant foods and 2. If necessary, supplement with magnesium.

When it comes to the best sources of magnesium on the planet, the winners are clearly in the plant kingdom. Based on the United States Department of Agriculture database, here are the champion food categories:[252]

- Beans
- Seeds
- Green leafy vegetables

Eat more of these foods and you are on the road to better magnesium levels.

However, dietary intake is not always adequate. Medical research suggests that if you have diabetes, your kidneys may be less able to retain magnesium.[253] Deficiency can result. Common medications like anti-ulcer and heartburn drugs known as proton pump inhibitors also tend to result in magnesium deficiency.[254] The generic names of these drugs end in "prazole" such as dex-lansoprazole (Dexilent®), esomeprazole (Nexium®), lansoprazole (Prevacid®), omeprazole (Prilosec®), pantoprazole (Protonix®), and rabeprazole (Aciphex®). But beware: The older generation of acid-blocking medications like ranitidine (Zantac®) and famotidine (Pepcid®) also put users at risk of low magnesium levels.[255]

Diuretics (water pills) are yet another class of drugs associated with magnesium losses. These medications are used to treat swelling as well as high blood pressure and heart failure. Examples of magnesium-robbing diuretics include hydrochlorothiazide (HCTZ), chlorthalidone, and furosemide (Lasix®). In short, if you have questions about your magnesium status, or merely want to take something for insurance, consider supplementation.

While at a recent conference, a health professional who knew of my magnesium advocacy approached me. He asked me which particular type of magnesium supplement I recommended. I told him I typically wasn't concerned whether a patient took magnesium chloride, magnesium gluconate, magnesium oxide, or any other form of magnesium, so long as they were keeping their blood magnesium levels up. (Of note, an insurance plan popular with many of my patients generally seems to cover magnesium oxide 400 mg pills, but no other magnesium sources.)

I then explained my rule of thumb. Start with your choice of magnesium supplement at a low level, gradually increase over days or weeks until your stools get too loose, then back off slightly. Yes, the main side effect of too much magnesium is loose stools. This laxative property of magnesium lies behind the age-old laxative uses of magnesium citrate and milk of magnesia.

The main group of people who consistently need to *avoid* magnesium are those with kidney problems. *If you have known kidney disease, do not take magnesium without a doctor's orders.* One other group that can get into problems are those who are taking some less commonly prescribed water pills.[256] These include: amiloride (Midamor®), spironolactone (Aldactone®), and triamterene (Dyrenium®). If you are taking one of these medications, you should generally avoid magnesium supplementation, unless instructed to do so by your doctor.

Here are some additional salient points about magnesium supplementation:[257]

- Supplementation with 300 – 400 mg of *elemental magnesium* appears necessary for some of magnesium's benefits such as blood pressure lowering.[258]

- For this reason, if you don't want to push your intake to

the point of bowel issues, then shoot for at least 300 mg of *elemental magnesium* daily.

- Realize that only a portion of any magnesium supplement is actually magnesium. For example, if a supplement bottle says each pill contains "500 mg of magnesium as magnesium oxide," you will only be getting about 300 mg of elemental magnesium per pill. The other 200 mg is made up of the "oxide" component.[259]

- Wondering how much elemental magnesium is found in common magnesium sources? Phillips' Milk of Magnesia® provides 500 mg of elemental magnesium in the form of magnesium hydroxide per tablespoon.

- Magnesium can adversely impact medication absorption. Susceptible drugs include thyroid medication, certain antibiotics, and bisphosphonates, medications used to treat osteoporosis. Medications in this latter class include alendronate (Fosamax®), etidronate (Didronel®), risedronate (Actonel®), and tiludronate (Skelid®). You can usually avoid absorption problems by taking the prescription drug at least two hours before you take your magnesium supplement. If you have questions about supplement and drug interactions, check with your pharmacist.

It's that time again. The choices are before you. Choose to either make a commitment to specific practices designed to promote dental health or increase your intake of magnesium. If you are really bold, why not do both?

35

DAY 21: BE HUMBLE

Today's Challenge: Reassess the lifestyle goals that you have set over the last 20 days, identify at least one area where you could be humbler, taking my counsel more seriously and making a larger commitment. Then put that broader commitment into practice for the rest of the program. (Examples: you have cut down on your coffee consumption, but you now decide to make a clean break with all caffeinated beverages; you have been walking 15 minutes per day, but want to boost that up to 30 minutes daily.)

I'M WRITING THIS CHAPTER while on a business trip. The work that brought me to this distant venue is completed, and I've settled down for an evening of writing. I've been making good progress; the only minor distraction has been an occasional whiff of a faint strange smell. However, I haven't lost focus due to that subtle odor. My writing has continued apace.

My wife, Sonja, who accompanied me on this trip had been out with some friends. She recently returned to the hotel room.

In our ensuing interaction, she notices something on my shoe. (Hours before, I had taken off my dress shoes and donned my more comfortable running shoes.) The strange smell is a mystery no longer. I realize that during my morning run I had planted one foot in a mass of excrement.

I'm obviously back to writing now. But I just finished most of the work of cleaning my shoe. A large portion of that task was completed in the bathroom, sitting on the side of the tub while leaning over the toilet. Using a Bic pen that I decided to sacrifice to the cause, I laboriously removed feces from every crevice of the sole.

Quite the humble picture. Your physician-author doing the most menial of tasks. Perhaps some of you think I should have just bagged both shoes and dumped them into one of the garbage cans flanking the hotel's main entrance!

But with this chapter's title in front of me, I couldn't help reflecting on the experience. To paraphrase a popular saying, "Excrement happens." But the bigger question is, what do we do when those undesirable events derail our life and plans? Now I think we would all agree, in the grand scheme of things, if a run-in with feces is the worst that life serves me, my life has been incredibly blessed. However, despite the unimpressive magnitude of today's mishap, I'm still captivated by the analogy (even if there's no more odor to remind me of the experience).

Think about it. I could have been fuming while doing that mundane task in the bathroom. *Why didn't that jerk clean up after his dog? How did I end up in a city that doesn't have stricter animal control laws?* Fortunately, my mind didn't go in any of those directions. I humbled myself and accepted my fate.

Would different circumstances have affected my reaction? If earlier today, during the conference I was attending, someone grabbed my leg and smeared feces all over the sole of my shoe, would I have responded differently?

If you really think about it, when bad things happen to us—whether in relationships, work, finances, or any other domain—we have only two basic postures from which to respond. I can be humble, accept that something bad happened to me, and focus on remedying my situation. Or I can be proud, nurturing the sense that my rights were violated, and focusing on putting something or someone in their place for the inconvenience, pain (or worse) that they have inflicted.

If someone cuts me off in traffic, or mistreats me at work, or doesn't respect me in a public venue, I can respond with anger, or with tears. Either way I'm saying that I deserve better. *This shouldn't happen to me. Don't they realize who I am? No one has the right to treat me that way.* On a certain level these are responses of pride. Now, I'm not saying that those reactions or responses are necessarily bad. Yes, in most contexts we associate negative connotations with *pride*. But anyone who has championed Black Pride, or Gay Pride, or Native Pride, was not embracing a cause that they perceived as negative. Instead, they most certainly had a positive motivation: perhaps to bolster themselves and others like them with a sense of value and acceptance.

Now I realize I'm already treading on dangerous ground, that of social justice. My intent is not to say that there aren't times to be angry with the status quo. On multiple occasions I've championed the rights of someone or a group who I believed was being mistreated. However, there's a Methuselah Factor price that we pay whenever we focus on things that make us angry, and that is because anger and hostility have been linked to worsened blood fluidity.[260]

However, if I don't focus on *my personal* rights, much of the grounds for anger is removed. The ancient scriptures had something to say along these lines. "I am under obligation [to help others]"[261] and "in humility count others more significant than yourselves."[262]

Realize that a humble spirit does not mean that we are content with passivity or that we need to be *doormats*. Jack Coulehan, MD, MPH has argued that "humility requires toughness and emotional resilience," being characterized by "unflinching self-awareness; empathic openness to others;" and gratitude for the privilege of helping those in need.[263] Hence, true humility has been defined as "the art of self-forgetfulness,"[264] which involves "not thinking less of ourselves but thinking of ourselves less."[265]

Because I've already alluded to racial inequality, there is another part of the puzzle we must consider. There is a growing body of literature that connects discrimination to poor cardiovascular outcomes. Specifically, there appears to be a connection between the stress of racial and/or gender discrimination, worsened inflammation in the body, and poorer blood fluidity.[266]

If you are the victim of discrimination, the research seems to put you in a difficult situation. If you focus on the violation of your rights, you impair your blood fluidity in the short term. However, if you avoid any attempt at making the situation better, you're dooming yourself and others to remain in an environment that impairs blood fluidity over the long term. Perhaps the solution has been best illustrated by civil rights champions in recent history like Martin Luther King, Nelson Mandela, and Mahatma Ghandi. These men were not known primarily for their ethnic pride, anger, or passion over their *personal* rights being trampled. Instead they were noted for a humility that blended self-forgetfulness with a steadfast purpose to help downtrodden peoples, even at their own expense.

Take up a just cause where you lose sight of self, where personal pride is laid aside, and you free yourself to experience gratitude on a higher level. If my focus is on how I've personally been mistreated, the springs of gratitude are blocked. It's hard to be happy or grateful when a selfish perspective leads you to dwell on how others are treated better then you, have more than you have, or are compensated better than you are. However, if I focus on helping others, even if there is still much headway to be made, I can rejoice with each small victory. And all this is extremely important when it comes to the Methuselah Factor. Medical research has begun to link gratitude to beneficial effects on blood fluidity.[267] Furthermore, true humility and gratitude can insulate against depression, which in turn has linkages with impaired hemorheology.[268]

Back to my morning run. Some of you might think I was too complacent. However, I really wasn't mad at the guy who didn't clean up after his dog (after all, it could have been a stray). And I didn't feel that the local municipality had violated my rights to walk in a feces-free city. As my day is winding down, I have a sense of gratitude for all that has happened today.

Embrace humility rather than pride, and you will react differently to obstacles. Ironically, a humble spirit may cause you to lose sight of personal affronts, but it may make you more aware of your need to champion causes that affect *others like you.*

Practicing Humility During Our Thirty-day Journey

Have you been humble enough to take my initial challenge from Day 1 and to truly "be bold"? Have you been willing to embrace key aspects of *The Methuselah Factor Diet and Lifestyle Program,* even if they didn't seem palatable on the surface? Have you been willing to go the extra mile? For example:

- When I challenged you to eat more beans and other plant

foods, did you commit to going on a total vegetarian diet for the remainder of the program?

- When I suggested cutting back on caffeine, have you eliminated it altogether from your lifestyle?
- When it came to my challenge to call the blood bank, did you go the extra mile and actually donate blood?

Let's dwell momentarily on this latter point. It seems that somewhere along the way, every medical student gets at least some exposure to medical history. For example, it is not uncommon for medical school teachers to remind their students how far their particular discipline—or the entire practice of medicine—has come. It was always in this context that I heard discussions about bloodletting, the practice that gave rise to the barber-surgeons of yesteryear. It was that practice, by the way, which has been implicated in the death of George Washington. Most historians agree that he had been bled to death.

However, if we cultivate humility (and a willingness to learn from the past), the history of bloodletting should cause us to pause, at least momentarily. Although bloodletting sounds barbaric, is it not reasonable to assume that a practice perpetuated for centuries would have *some* benefits? As expressed in Chapters 8 and 15, most of us would be helped by parting with limited amounts of our blood—at least occasionally. I'm not advocating the revitalization of the barber-surgeon career path; my emphasis, instead, is on a practice calculated to not only improve your hemorheology but also to help your neighbors: blood donation.

You should have, by this time in the program, called your local blood bank or blood donation center. If you do nothing else today—make plans to donate blood before the end of this week. Be humble enough to accept my encouragement over all your well-intentioned objections.

If you've already donated blood during this thirty-day journey, then look back over the previous chapter titles and the target behaviors that you have listed in Figure 15. Where could you be doing better? Resolve to be bold, but also humble enough to more fully implement my advice from previous days of this program.

Today's challenge is a one-time task. Choose just one target behavior that you have committed yourself to (sometime between Day 1 and 20) and enhance it. For example, if on Day 9 you committed to doing resistance exercise once per week, why not twice weekly? Next, indicate, on Figure 15, how you're refining that target behavior. In the case of our example, you would erase or white out the number "1" and put a "2" in the blank for Day 9. It would then read: *Do resistance exercise _2_ times per week*. Finally, make two other changes on that same Figure 15. First, mark an "X" in the box for Day 21 under the column for this chapter (identified as *Chapter 35*, with the stated goal to "Improve at least one of your previous target behaviors"). Second, put an "X" in all the rest of the boxes in that column (corresponding to Days 22 to 30).

Those changes in Figure 15 will make it clear that you need to execute today's challenge only once. Thank you, in advance, for being humble enough to embrace more broadly the principles that we've been studying and to ramp up your program for the home stretch.

36

DAY 22: EAT, FAST

Today's Challenge: Plan to engage in some type of fasting on a daily or, at least, weekly basis.

PUNCTUATION MATTERS. LEAVE OUT the comma in today's chapter title and you'll think I'm urging you to wolf down your food. Quite the contrary. Today I'm challenging you to eat at appropriate meal times, but then fast (avoid all caloric intake) between those meals.

Years ago, I had the privilege of being selected as a speaker for the National Wellness Conference, in Steven's Point, Wisconsin. Perhaps the most memorable part of that conference was the opportunity to personally interact with another one of the lecturers, Dr. Lester Breslow. Although not of physically imposing stature, Dr. Breslow was a giant in the field of public health. His resume included Dean of UCLA's School of Public Health, Director of the California State Department of Public Health, and President of the American Public Health Association.

During the conference, I enjoyed Breslow's fascinating

account of how he launched the "Human Population Laboratory" in California's Alameda County. That project, started in the 1960s, generated some of the earliest data linking healthy lifestyle to longevity. During my Masters' training in Public Health, Breslow's data from Alameda County was featured front and center.

However, in my personal interaction with Breslow, I was preoccupied with one burning question. I had read a number of Breslow's papers and knew that when he initially studied the Alameda County residents he had found that *eating between meals* was associated with dying sooner. However, years later, some of Breslow's younger colleagues had sought to minimize the importance of this practice, originally popularized as one of Breslow's seven pillars of longevity. So, I posed the question: "What do you think? Is there really a connection between snacking and mortality?" Dr. Breslow was unequivocal. Although he didn't disparage his colleagues, it was clear he felt some of them hadn't seen the full picture yet. *Fasting between meals was most definitely a key to longevity.*

Dr. Breslow's posture, articulated at that meeting many years ago, has now been given further validation by the science of hemorheology. For example, intermittent fasting has been demonstrated to decrease levels of proinflammatory and/or blood-fluidity-impairing compounds like interleukin 6, homocysteine, C-reactive protein, and total white blood cell count.[269,270,271]

To get the full advantage of this thirty-day program I want you to include some form of fasting in the week or so that remains. How then do you fast? There are a number of ways to implement today's challenge. Before looking at some specific examples of fasting, some definitions are in order. Tatiana Moro and colleagues provided some useful working definitions in their 2016 research article:[272]

- "In humans, fasting is achieved by ingesting little to no

food or caloric beverages for periods that typically range from 12 h[ours] to 3 weeks."

- "Fasting is distinct from caloric restriction (CR), in which daily caloric intake is chronically reduced by up to 40 %, but meal frequency is maintained."

- "IF [Intermittent Fasting] is defined by a complete or partial restriction in energy intake (between 50 and 100 % restriction of total daily energy intake) on 1–3 days per week or a complete restriction in energy intake for a defined period during the day that extends the overnight fast."

Moro and associates point out that the most studied form of fasting comes from the Muslim spiritual tradition. Ramadan fasting involves abstinence from all eating and drinking from dawn to sunset during the month of Ramadan (which, being based on a lunar calendar, varies from our current 12-month time frame). Other spiritual fasting traditions are cited by the University of California, San Diego's Dr. Ruth Patterson and colleagues in their review of intermittent fasting. Among these they mention that: "Seventh-day Adventists often consume their last of two daily meals in the afternoon, which results in a long nighttime fasting period that may be biologically important." However, many other fasting regimens have been popularized, many without any religious connections. For example, Patterson's team cited Mosley and Spencer's best-selling book, *The Fast Diet*, which promoted marked caloric restriction for two days a week with normal eating during the remaining five days.

You can fulfill today's challenge by implementing any one of the fasts that I've just mentioned. However, for the purposes of this chapter, I will even allow you to implement a strategy of caloric restriction. Here are examples of some different ways you could embrace today's challenge:

217

1. No caloric intake after 3 PM for the rest of your thirty-day program

2. Skipping suppers

3. One or more days per week of juice-only fasting

4. Excluding specific foods for the rest of your program

5. No eating between meals

6. One or more days per week where you fast totally (no caloric intake) or severely reduce intake (e.g., to no more than 500 calories per day) [Beware: If you take medications or have other health issues, I discourage total fasting unless you are working with a health professional]

7. Implementing the leaf-stem-and-flower fast for one or more days per week

Most of the seven options above are self-explanatory. However, let me give you some additional background and explanation that may help you come up with a viable personal game plan.

For years I have guided patients on intermittent fasting regimens. My initial interest began when working with type 2 diabetes. We found that several days of water-only fasting in a supervised medical setting would typically result in dramatic blood sugar decreases. In one series of patients we studied, the majority were able to discontinue insulin and remain off their shots when they went back to eating, all with better blood sugars.[273] We also had excellent results with high blood pressure, seeing patients dramatically lower their pressure—and keep it down—thanks to a jump start with a water-only fast. Impressive results with diabetes and high blood pressure were not findings unique to our practice.[274]

However, such an approach had its challenges. We had to

ensure that a patient's electrolytes (blood minerals) were acceptable at the outset of the fast and then reassess those levels if the fast was continued for any significant duration (in most cases, more than three to five days). Before they began a water-only fast, we had to adjust patients' medications, especially those affecting blood sugar and blood pressure. As the fast progressed, further medication changes were sometimes necessary. We also learned that some patients could not tolerate a total fast. Among this group were those prone to digestive problems like stomach ulcers or irritation (gastritis) and gastroesophageal reflux disease (the common cause of heartburn). These individuals seemed to do best if they ate something to help buffer their stomach acid.

It was in this latter context that we found a particular low-calorie diet to be especially effective. We called it the leaf-stem-and-flower fast. You have already been exposed to this approach in Chapter 33. You may recall that on such a fast a person is able to eat all the leaf, stem, and flower vegetables that he or she desires. Remember also: these vegetables tend to be very low in something called glycemic index, which means they generally don't raise blood sugar much. Furthermore, these foods are generally very low in calories, allowing a person to eat a significant volume and still markedly decrease his or her caloric intake.

On an additional note, those leaf-stem-and-flower foods are very low in fat. This is noteworthy when considering the Methuselah Factor. For years, researchers have noted that higher fat diets tend to worsen blood fluidity by elevating the activity of pro-clotting compounds like Factor VII and Factor VIII.[275]

This observation is also relevant when we consider option 4 in our "menu" of fasting strategies, "Excluding specific foods for the rest of your program." Some might be tempted to avoid most carbohydrates and follow an Atkins-type diet. If you are not familiar with such dietary strategies, they generally involve eating relatively large amounts of protein and fat compared to carbohydrates. Although a fast or diet where you can eat liberal amounts of cheese, meat, bacon and eggs might sound appealing—and the research does show it can help with weight loss—I advise against such an approach on several grounds. First, are the connections we have just observed between higher fat diets and worsened blood fluidity. But beyond that, low carbohydrate diets can produce unusual stresses on organs like the kidneys, bones, and intestines.[276,277]

To illustrate the potential dangers of a low carbohydrate, Atkins-type diet, a team of Japanese gastroenterologists (intestinal specialists) recently reported the case of a 38-year-old physician.[278] Two years earlier this doctor had adopted an Atkins diet and lost about 13 pounds. He stayed on the low carb plan and was able to keep the weight off. However, he began to have bloody stools and was ultimately diagnosed with a serious bowel disorder known as ulcerative colitis (UC). His doctors placed him on a "plant-based/semi-vegetarian diet." The result was remission of his UC without any need for medication.

My recommendation is if you are leaving out certain foods to meet today's challenge that you choose foods that are generally unhealthy on other grounds: certain dessert choices, soft drinks (if you haven't already eliminated them), red meat, cheese, etc. Unless you have a known food sensitivity don't choose whole grains, beans, fruits, or vegetables, as the food categories you eliminate.

I think you have the idea. Implement some type of fasting for the rest of your program. This is another important aspect of *The Methuselah Factor Diet and Lifestyle Program*, and another important tool to help you optimize your blood fluidity.

37

DAY 23: IDENTIFY YOUR STRESSORS

Today's Challenge: Identify your stressors, paying attention to each of the following domains: physical, mental, emotional, social, and spiritual. (Tomorrow we will begin looking at strategies to deal with these stressors.)

BALLISTIC MISSILE THREAT INBOUND TO HAWAII. SEEK IMMEDIATE SHELTER. THIS IS NOT A DRILL

WIDESPREAD PANIC SWEPT OVER Hawaii when, on Saturday, January 13, 2018, the message above appeared on hundreds of thousands of cellphones and countless TV screens. What the world and the residents of Hawaii *soon* knew was that message was in error. There was no missile threat. However, *soon* was not *soon enough* for most Hawaiians. It took a full 38 minutes before an official retraction was widely disseminated.

Alia Wong's brother was living in Hawaii during the scare. His panicked Saturday morning phone call alerted Alia to the pandemonium playing out in our Westernmost state. The next day, Alia penned the following account in *The Atlantic*:[279]

> People across the state were terrified. Many assumed they would die, but sought shelter anyway. They took cover in mall bathrooms, bathtubs, drug stores—even a storm drain. Hawaii has very few shelters, and houses with basements are rare. There were reports of people speeding down highways and running red lights to reunite with family members. Others called one another to say "I love you" one last time.
>
> ...It took officials 38 minutes to announce their mistake, and to confirm that the warning had been a false alarm. Those 38 minutes were the 38 worst minutes of many Hawaii residents' lives. And they were just as horrifying for people outside of Hawaii who, like me, felt helpless as they contended with the prospect of never seeing their loved ones again.

How could something go so terribly wrong? Over the hours, days, and weeks that followed different accounts circulated. Initial reports described an employee who inadvertently sent out a true alert message instead of a test alert. Later accounts described a confused employee who genuinely thought there was missile crisis when the alert trigger was pulled. Regardless of what actually happened the facts are clear: there was no real danger, but thousands were terribly *stressed out*.

This account offers some very important insights into stress. Many people think that stress is caused by something or someone other than themselves, like a false missile alarm. However, the concept of stress is a bit more complicated. Scientists use the term *stressors* to refer to the things, often outside ourselves, that upset our equilibrium. Stressors can confront us on any level of our existence: physical, mental, emotional, social, or spiritual. In the Hawaiian example, the stressor was the false alarm.

However, the way we react to those stressors is called the stress response. It is this response that determines how a given stressor or stressors affect us physiologically.

There is no report of any comatose patient in Hawaii having any stress response to that January 13 false alarm. It is possible some severely depressed patients breathed a sigh of relief when they received the notices; *now I won't have to take my own life,* they could have reasoned. An estranged wife in California might have been encouraged that the threats from her Honolulu-based ex might finally be coming to an end. Granted, some of these scenarios might seem a bit morbid, but here's the point: people and events can confront us as stressors but it is up to us, at least on some level, to influence whether or not those things *stress us out.*

The plot thickens when you realize that in stress science circles they sometimes add Greek prefixes to the mix. *Eu* refers to good while *dis* refers to bad (think *eu*phoria as opposed to *dis*ease). Armed with this information you might be able to figure out how I like to define a *eustressor.* Although the research literature may feature somewhat different definitions for this and related terms, I find the following conceptualization helpful.

Eustressors are things that we perceive as desirable, but nonetheless require our bodies to adapt. An example would be notice of winning the lottery. Most people would be overjoyed with such an announcement. But as good as the initial perception is, there is still a stress response. I was reminded years ago that such a stress response can, at times, be overwhelming. A close relative of one of my grad school teachers died within days of learning that she won the lottery!

On the other hand, I define *distressors* as things confronting us which we view as undesirable. When most people think of stressors and the stress response, they're thinking of such distressors.

We can also apply our Greek prefixes to the *stress response*. A stressor, whether perceived as a eustressor or a distressor, can cause either a eustress response or a distress response. In the case of the lottery winner, the eustressor caused severe distress. But how about deadlines? Are they eustressors or distressors? Do they cause a eustress response or a distress response? It, really, depends. Although a deadline might be perceived as a distressor, if it helps you complete an important task in a timely manner, the result might be a sense of accomplishment—eustress, if you will. Consequently, when most people speak of eustressors, they often use words like *challenge*, rather than *stress* per se.

Stress is an inevitable part of living—in good times and in bad. The key for each of us is to try to thrive in the midst of our eustressors and distressors. When our internal self-talk and perceptions help us maintain an even keel, we keep our stress system dialed down. This helps to optimize our Methuselah Factor. In the world of stress, it is not so much what happens to you but, rather, your perception of it that largely determines the effects on your blood fluidity and overall health.[280]

Over the next three days we are going to take a careful look at stress and stressors. The relationships are important because, as we've already been seeing throughout this book, stress hormones are generally deleterious when it comes to our hemorheology. For example, mental stress makes your platelets more likely to aggregate or stick together.[281,282] Sure, if a tiger is about to attack you, you want your body to move immediately into *fight or flight* mode.

And you want your platelets to be stickier so your blood will quickly clot if you sustain a non-life-threatening injury. However, if someone cuts you off in traffic, or you deal with sustained stressors in the home or workplace, then those same stress hormones will not serve you very well. Your Methuselah Factor will suffer.

Today's assignment is relatively easy. I want you to take some time to identify your stressors. What things right now are challenging you? I've made the process easier by providing Figure 19. That figure lists five domains of stressors: physical, mental, emotional, social, and spiritual. For each one I give some tangible examples. Your challenge for today is to simply fill out the fourth column.

Once you've completed the chart in Figure 19, you have finished today's challenge. (Just as you did with the one-time task for Chapter 35, upon completion of Figure 19, check off all the boxes in the column corresponding to Chapter 37 in Figure 15.) Over the next two days we'll look at strategies to deal with the stressors that you've identified.

	FIGURE 19	Five Domains of Stressors	
Domain	**Example of Type of Stressor**	**Specific Illustrations of Common Stressors**	**My Personal Stressors in this Domain**
Physical	Temperature	– My husband keeps the bedroom temperature colder than I like	
Mental	Financial and Occupational Issues	– Balancing your budget	
Emotional	Emotional Response to Environmental Risks	– Fears of natural disasters (flooding during Gulf Coast hurricane season, fires during fire season in Western U.S.)	
Social	Relationships	– Tensions at home – Bullying at work	
Spiritual	Areas of Meaning and Purpose	– What is my real calling in life? – Is there a God, Creator, or other higher power?	

38

DAY 24: ELIMINATE SOME STRESSORS

Today's Challenge: Identify at least one stressor that you plan to eliminate, then each day for the rest of this program begin making steps in that direction.

MY FRIEND RICK SAID that it was a terrible commute. It wasn't just the one-hour drive nor even the heavy traffic. No, it was the other drivers. More than once he'd been on the receiving end of road rage.

Rick never asked me for help dealing with his stressful commute, but one day he announced the solution. He had moved to within five minutes of his workplace.

Rick had employed one of the most effective strategies for dealing with a stressor. *He had removed it.* Of course, we can't remove every stressor. And even if a stressor can be removed, it is not always easy or optimal to do so.

I realize this may sound like a strange topic to be addressing during the final week of our journey. After all, if I were challenging you to move, it would likely entail far more than you could surround before your thirty-day program was finished. However, there are many stressors that are far simpler to address than removing an onerous commute. In order to eliminate stressors, we must first identify them. That was yesterday's assignment. Today we turn our attention to selecting one or more stressors that we could eliminate, often by a single decisive action.

For example, let's say that, when you filled out Figure 19, you identified a major physical stressor, your weight. Perhaps you feel that you're carrying an extra 60 pounds. Now, you might be thinking, *Yes, Dr. DeRose I'm ready to have someone remove those excess pounds*. However, that option is not at our disposal. Instead you'll have to drill down a bit and ask some other questions. How did I gain those extra 60 pounds? Why can't I lose the extra weight?

Look back at Figure 19. You may or may not have identified other *related stressors* when it came to the mental or environmental domains. However, it is likely that there are things in both these domains (and others) that are contributing to your weight.

For example, upon reflection, you might realize that you are likely to overeat, eat between meals, or make poor food choices when feeling down or depressed. With this in mind, you could *remove* all the junk food from your home, so that if you're feeling down there won't be any bad options easily accessible. If that's not viable (perhaps you share a home with others who have different lifestyle priorities), then you can *remove* the possibility of bad dietary choices by going to a food-less venue when feeling depressed. For example, you could head over to the health club or your local place of worship, presuming those are both food-free zones. (Of interest, research has linked faith community attendance with better adherence to healthy lifestyle practices.)[283]

If, instead, your main high-risk scenario for overeating occurs in your living room when sitting in your easy chair and watching TV, you could simply rearrange your living room. If *removing* the TV is too bold a step, you could *remove* the easy chair and put an exercise bicycle in its place. (Most people find it more difficult to munch on chips or down ice cream while riding a stationary cycle, than sitting in a plush chair.)

When it comes to removing your stressors, then, you are really focusing on at least two things: 1. The stressor you want to eliminate, and 2. The factors that may be contributing to the distress connected with the stressor.

Over the years I've helped many patients and groups address their stressors. If you are looking for a couple of engaging video presentations on the topic, feel free to pick up a copy of my *Changing Bad Habits for Good* DVD.[284] I also have a free, online thirty-day YouTube series that provides additional insights on how to remove stressors on Day 24 of that series. Although the YouTube series is especially themed to address diabetes and/or high blood pressure, I cover similar topics to this book's chapters in the daily videos.[285] For example, Day 24 in the video series bears the same title as this chapter, "Eliminate Some Stressors."

I'm not expecting you to rely on either the DVD or on-line series in order to be successful with today's challenge. Therefore, let me give you a few high points from those presentations that will make it clearer how to identify—and remove—susceptible stressors, especially if your own behaviors are stressing you out. Perhaps the best way to do this is by calling your attention to the following figure.

FIGURE 20A	The A, B, Cs of Removing Behavioral Stressors	
Antecedents	Behaviors	Consequences
	Arriving Late for Work	

In Figure 20A, we have listed a possible stressor, a behavior: *arriving late for work*. The key to removing this behavior lies in part with understanding the setting in which it occurs. The setting is sometimes described in terms of "antecedents," literally, that which comes before. You can hone in on high risk antecedents by asking the journalist's 5 Ws: Who, What, Where, When, and Why. In other words, certain people, places, and things can put you at high risk for running late.

Later in this chapter I'll be asking you to fill in Figure 21. Right now, I'll walk you through Figures 20B and 20C to help you understand one of the more efficient ways to, ultimately, fill out Figure 21.

Figure 20B lists some possible antecedents that you might have identified, each of which can predispose you to running late. Once you've identified the antecedents, your job becomes easier. You now know where the battle lines are drawn. Your task is come up with a strategy to remove the antecedents. Let's look at them one by one.

FIGURE 20B	The A, B, Cs of Removing Behavioral Stressors	

Antecedents	Behaviors	Consequences
- Not knowing what to wear - Traffic delays - Early morning arguments with significant other	Arriving Late for Work	

Not knowing what to wear. If you find this to be a periodic morning stressor, there is an easy way to remove it. Simply pick out your clothes and shoes the night before. Now, I realize this seems obvious (and I'm really not trying to insult you). However, some of our stressors are relatively easy to address if we just recognize where the battle lies.

Traffic delays. Obviously, this is not something that you can remove. However, many of you can remove this from being a distressor. How? Simply shift your schedule early enough that even a major traffic delay would not scuttle your plans to be on time. Getting up 30 minutes earlier and walking out the door even 15 minutes earlier may be all that's needed for many of you. Granted, some of you live in locations with only one major thoroughfare to work. It may be impossible in that scenario to get up early enough to cover all contingencies (like total closure of an interstate from a multicar accident). However, you get the idea.

Early morning arguments with your significant other. If you share a home or an apartment with others, there is always a chance for emotions to flare just at the time you should be walking out the door. However, just as you can set your clothes aside the night before, so you can set aside the fuel for arguments each evening. The Apostle Paul said: "let not the sun go down upon your wrath."[286] In other words, address your anger before retiring for the night. It will help you sleep better, and you'll be less likely to awaken in a polarized environment.

When the Antecedents are Hard to Identify

So far everything may seem straight forward. But if you've jumped ahead and have already begun working on Figure 21, there's a chance you're having difficulty identifying your antecedents. Here's where Figure 20C comes into play. In this example, we're looking at a different behavioral stressor. This time it's your cigarette smoking. Now, not everyone is mentally stressed out by his or her own smoking. But you say that you are. You know it is messing up your Methuselah Factor, your chronic cough is worsening, and your spouse is nagging you about the habit. You're ready to quit, but you need some additional insights and motivation. You sense tapping into stuff about antecedents may help you, but you're stumped as to what to list.

Although you can't tell from Figure 20C, it's a figure I began filling out using the third column dedicated to *consequences*. Identifying negative consequences can help to motivate you to change. (That's what you did when you mentally listed smoking's deleterious effects on your Methuselah Factor, your cough, and your spousal relationship.) However, identifying *positive consequences* of what you are now labeling a *bad behavior* can give you insights into your high-risk antecedents. Think about it this way: if your bad habits were not doing something "good" for you, you would have stopped those behaviors long ago.

When it comes to your work, on Figure 21, you are welcome to list the negative consequences of the behavior that you want to change. Keeping those negatives in plain view can help to motivate you and to maintain your resolve. However, especially when you are at a loss to identify antecedents, make sure that you also list the positive consequences, or benefits, of your undesirable behaviors. That's what I've done for you in Figure 20C.

FIGURE 20C	The A, B, Cs of Removing Behavioral Stressors	
Antecedents	**Behaviors**	**Consequences**
	Smoking Cigarettes	Positive
1. Feeling Stressed		1. Helps me feel relaxed
2. Feeling underappreciated at work		2. Gives me a sense of reward

In Figure 20C, you began by filling out the third column, which is dedicated to consequences. There you first identified that smoking helps you relax. This should give you a window on high-risk antecedents. Think about it. When do you feel a need to relax? I've listed *feeling stressed* for you in the corresponding antecedent column. Now you have a better idea where you must direct special efforts. When feeling under stress on the job, you will likely have the desire to smoke. What to do about it? You can't remove all feelings of stress, but you can *remove* cigarettes and lighters from your environment (your office and car). Better yet, do something active that removes you, or keeps you, from the environment where you used to smoke. If in the past you would head out the door for a smoke in the parking lot, now head to the inside stairwell where no smoking is allowed. Walk up and down your building's three flights of stairs until the urge dissipates. And, yes, exercise is a powerful dissipator of stressed emotions.

I listed another positive consequence of smoking in Figure 20C. You say it gives you a sense of reward. Perhaps you just finished a major project or task at home. (It could be anything, simple or complex: doing the laundry, cooking dinner, fixing a stubborn toilet or repainting the entire interior.) You're impressed with the good job that you've done, and a cigarette seems the perfect way to reward yourself. If you were to reflect on it, this seems especially important because, based on your previous experience, no one at home will likely commend you for the job you just completed. So, again, you can't remove the sense of accomplishment when you've done a job well; nor can you necessarily force people to thank you for your hard work (although it might not hurt to ask). However, you can *remove* the expectation of a cigarette as a reward. Why not come up with another way to reward yourself? Make a quick trip to a store (preferably one that does not sell cigarettes) and reward yourself with something that will help you complete a similar task next time. Perhaps it is a kitchen implement, a new spice, or a plumbing tool.

Remember, you will work Figure 21 *backwards*, just like we did

234

in Figure 20C, if you want to use the positive consequences of a behavioral stressor to provide insights into important antecedents. In other words, fill out those positive consequences first. Then go back to the antecedents and identify settings where you will likely be looking for the positive consequences that your undesirable behavior has been providing. Then either remove those antecedents or remove other aspects of those settings that might set you up to fail.

That's your task for today. Notice that in Figure 21 you can list up to three different behavioral stressors. Feel free to list as many as three in the table. However, commit to addressing at least one over the remaining week of your *Methuselah Factor Diet and Lifestyle Program*.

FIGURE 21	The A, B, Cs of Removing Behavioral Stressors	
Antecedents	Behaviors	Consequences

39

DAY 25: HARNESS SOME STRESSORS

Today's Challenge: Identify something in your life that is stressful and come up with a strategy to make that stressor an advantage rather than a disadvantage.

FOR OVER 16 YEARS I've had the privilege of serving as host of American Indian Living Radio.[287] In that capacity I've recorded hundreds of interviews that have aired weekly on some 170 stations. As you can imagine, I've received quite an education talking with many accomplished and fascinating guests who have joined me on the broadcast. My recent interview with Patrick Anderson, JD, was no exception.

Patrick has a fascinating background. He grew up challenged by a host of what experts call "adverse childhood experiences." As summarized in a recent scientific publication, "Adverse childhood experiences (ACEs) encompass any acts of commission or omission by a parent or other caregiver that result in harm, potential for harm or threat of harm to a child in the first 18 years of life, even if harm is not the intended result."[288] Such ACEs include "psychological, physical, or sexual abuse; violence against mother; or living with household members who were substance abusers, mentally ill or suicidal, or ever imprisoned."[289]

The research suggests that such rearing would have predisposed Patrick to a lifetime of physical, emotional, and mental health challenges including alcoholism, drug abuse, anxiety, depression, interpersonal and self-directed violence, heart disease, cancer, and asthma.[290] Yet here was Patrick sitting in front of me, seeming to be thriving. He was the CEO of a Native corporation, a graduate of Princeton University and the University of Michigan Law School. Even though his law degree was awarded some 40 years ago, he didn't show any evidence of cognitive decline; he was articulate and insightful, recalling details of numerous research studies by memory.

What Patrick communicated in his interview was the product of years of scientific research and personal reflection. He hypothesized, in essence, that the very factors that threaten to undermine our life and health can, instead, be harnessed to help us thrive.

For example, Patrick reviewed the research that connected ACEs with substance abuse. He then said that if someone knows that they are predisposed to use a drug to alter their brain chemistry, they can put their energies into improving their brain chemistry but with healthy stimuli. But his insights became most poignant when he segued to the example of cigarette smoking.

The essence of his argument was this: smokers will turn to nicotine dozens of times per day to get a quick brain "hit." If someone is predisposed to smoking, perhaps they need to engage in something multiple times per day that provides some of the "benefits" of smoking but without all the side effects. Among the strategies

Patrick discussed were harnessing the power of two conceptually simple behaviors: positive affirmations and smiling. We'll talk more about these shortly. However, for now, it is important to note that Patrick was focusing my radio listeners on what has been termed "positive psychology." Such a focus is also especially relevant for us as we near the conclusion of our thirty-day program. The reasons are myriad, but consider two:

1. Research indicates that the balance of our stress hormone system can be upset by adverse childhood experiences, as well as on-going present stressors.[291,292] We have already seen that abnormalities in this stress system can predispose to Methuselah Factor abnormalities.

2. Past and present stressors that we are incapable of removing or changing continue to have ongoing effects. We thus need to embrace strategies to help us thrive in the face of these stressors.

The Positive Psychology Movement

Nearly four decades ago, when I began my medical studies, the emphasis in the mental health arena was on disease and dysfunction. We learned theories about why patients developed psychiatric problems. We were taught about medications and counselling techniques that could be used to help these conditions. However, no one talked much about how patients could help themselves by using positive thinking. The same negative bias seems to creep into our discussions of stress. Let me illustrate.

When Dr. Greg Steinke, Nurse Practitioner Trudie Li and I, in our book, *Thirty Days to Natural Blood Pressure Control*, tackled the topic of stress, we shared one of my favorite stress illustrations. We painted the picture of you being confronted, in your own bedroom, by an apparently ravenous lion. In the illustration, the lion served as the tangible personification of a stressor.

When I've used that illustration with live audiences, I've asked participants to strategize ways to deal with the potentially life-threating situation. Among the responses I've chronicled are:

- Playing dead
- Shooting the lion
- Fighting the lion
- Trying to escape

However, one of the least common answers is *befriend the lion.* Yes, our bias is clearly to try to avoid stressors, especially if they are distressing. But it seems we've forgotten something that we were supposed to learn in grade school P.E. class: the only way you get stronger is by being stressed. Instead of getting rid of the lion in our bedrooms, if we befriend him, we can reap some impressive gains.

Illness Acceptance and Optimism Help Us Overcome Chronic Stressors

HIV infection. Inflammatory bowel disease. Progressive arthritis. These and hundreds of other chronic disease diagnoses are made multiple times daily in thousands of hospitals and clinics throughout the world.

That chronic diseases exist does not surprise us; however, what is surprising is how different people respond to being diagnosed with a chronic illness—and the lifetime of chronic stress such a diagnosis may entail. While some experience depression and introversion, others experience what is termed *posttraumatic growth.*

The analogy applies to any stressors that come into our life. When we face difficulties, our responses could be graphed on a

240

continuum. On one extreme are feelings of depression and overload, on the other extreme are gratitude and growth.

I recently ran into Jean at a social venue. We had been classmates many years before, but it was immediately obvious that things were far different than the last time we crossed paths several years ago. Jean was her usual upbeat self, but her wig and thinner frame provided clues of significant life changes.

Her husband, Otto, told me about Jean's cancer diagnosis and her ongoing chemotherapy. But then he said something surprising, "Four of our friends have been diagnosed with cancer this year. Although we sorrow with them, we've also been reminded that things could be much worse. Jean has a far better prognosis than several of our friends."

As I reflected on that conversation I was impressed with the foundations of gratitude. Even in very difficult situations, we can find reasons to be thankful. Yes, our gratitude might be focused on how much worse our situation could be. However, we can also give thanks for positive blessings, like supportive relationships and specific material benefits (such as access to adequate food and shelter).

We have already observed that gratitude appears to be associated, both directly and indirectly, with better blood fluidity. In view of this, awareness of life's stressors/challenges can provide opportunities to cultivate gratitude.

Indeed, when researchers look at what distinguishes those who experience posttraumatic growth and those who are overwhelmed, several factors emerge. Thriving, resilience, and growth are associated with:[293]

- Acceptance of one's situation (in contrast to denial)
- Stronger social support networks

- Optimism, including expectations of future growth
- Spirituality

Self-Affirmation and Smiling

The topic of optimism brings us back to Patrick Anderson's observations. He has advocated utilizing self-affirmation and smiling to help us thrive even while facing serious past or present stressors.

Try it some time. When you feel stressed, smile. When stressors seem to be coming at you from all sides, try some positive affirmations like "I can handle this," or "The Creator made me to succeed," or "My loved ones have confidence in me."

Several years ago, a medical journal featured an article with a captivating title, *Grin and Bear It: The Influence of Manipulated Facial Expression on the Stress Response.*[294] In it, researchers Kraft and Pressman from the University of Kansas shared results on 170 subjects who took part in a carefully designed smiling intervention. They found that smiling decreased the mental and emotional impact of a stressful task and resulted in less stress hormone-related effects (as manifested by lower heart rates).

Another fascinating paper was recently published by Michael Lewis of Cardiff University in the United Kingdom. Lewis looked at the effects of Botox injections on emotions. When Botox was used to decrease wrinkle lines associated with frowning, mood improved. However, when crow's feet (or *laughter lines*) were targeted, smiling was impaired and patients experienced a rise in depression scores.[295]

The messages couldn't be clearer. Get stress to work for you. When feeling under pressure, see it as a call to smile—and notify your face to act the part.

Patrick Anderson's other tool, self-affirmation, can be defined as a process "induced by reflecting upon important values, attributes, or social relations."[296] In a study designed to promote better blood pressure control through medication adherence, self-affirmation techniques and other strategies designed to encourage a positive outlook (when combined with instruction) were all found to foster better medication compliance than did education alone.[297] Specifically, the self-affirmation approach involved asking patients "to remember their core values and proud moments in their lives" when confronted by situations where they found it difficult to take their medications. Other studies have shown that similar self-affirmation practices can improve receptivity to other behavioral interventions.[298]

The bottom line is that self-affirmation can help us make better decisions when faced with life's stressors. It can also help foster a positive outlook even in difficult times. Indeed, cultivating a positive mind-set can help us avoid becoming overly stressed.

As noted, one way we can befriend stressors in general is to use an awareness of their presence to lead us to tap into positive sources like cultivating gratitude, self-affirmation, or smiling. In other words, feeling stressed is not a cue to slide into depression or inactivity, but rather to focus on positive mental skills. However, we can also befriend specific stressors—taking the very things that seek to overwhelm us and turning them into a blessing.

Dealing with a Disruptive Alarm Clock

Although some people seem to thrive when given time challenges and deadlines, others seem to wither under the pressure. However, the reality exists: some things in life have to be done in a timely manner.

Could you reperceive your assessment of deadlines? What would happen if you started looking at the clock as your friend, challenging you to accomplish a certain amount in a given period of time? Actually, one of the main differences between something

243

that stresses you out and serves as a helpful challenge is, simply, your self-talk. In other words, what you tell yourself about a stressor has the power to transform it from something that promotes distress to a factor that fosters eustress, satisfaction, and accomplishment.

Furthermore, the clock can stress us in other ways. For example, sharing a room with someone on a different work schedule can be stressful. Perhaps you have plenty of time if you roll out of bed by 6AM. Your sleeping partner, however, must arise by 4. How do you relate to that daily 4 AM alarm?

You actually have a number of choices. Sure, based on yesterday's discussion, you could simply avoid having to hear the alarm clock stressor by moving to another room in your house or apartment. However, if you want to stay in your bedroom together, you might ask the question: *How can I get this stressor to work for me?* In other words, instead of getting frustrated and stressed every time you hear that alarm, try coming up with some scenario where that alarm clock will work in your favor.

For example, are there any benefits you might reap by rising earlier? Perhaps your habitual 6 AM waking time is fine for your normal routine, but maybe you realize that you are not getting enough exercise. What would happen if you shifted your wake-up time a couple hours earlier and then started using that dusty home exercise equipment early each morning?

You get the idea. Look at the stressors in your life. First, see them as a call to embrace positive psychology strategies. But don't stop there; see if there are actual ways to get the stressors to work for you. It may not be a disruptive alarm clock, but it could be a disruptive person at work. Get to know the person who is stressing you out. Put yourself in their shoes and try to befriend them. You might be surprised by the transformation in you—and them.

40

DAY 26: SCRUTINIZE YOUR SUPPLEMENTS

Today's Challenge: Take careful inventory of any herbs, nutrients, or other supplements that you use regularly. Eliminate any that you are not certain are helping your blood fluidity and health in general.

IN MY EXPERIENCE, MOST people who share stories about their forays into the great outdoors speak of the benefits of such excursions: reconnecting with nature, de-stressing away from their typical urban surroundings, etc. However, on that particular day in my medical office, Renee had anything but positive stories to share when it came to her recent backpacking trip.

Renee and four friends had hiked a couple of days into some beautiful backcountry wilderness. It was then that the nightmare unfolded. Being a serious backpacker, Renee had packed exactly what she needed for the ten-day excursion, so when she opened up her evening rations, she struggled only for a few seconds about what to do. The entrée didn't taste very good. But she had never purchased this item before, and with only so many calories to sustain her on her journey, she felt obligated to eat something that she would have discarded had she been home. It was not until several hours later that Renee realized her mistake.

Even as morning began to dawn, there didn't seem to be any end in sight to the vomiting and diarrhea that had plagued Renee all night. She was exhausted. Her main task was struggling to keep down sips of water to ward off dehydration. As she and her friends sized up the options, there didn't appear to be many good ones. Renee was too weak to continue, and she also didn't have the energy to return to their vehicles. They collectively decided that Renee would spend the next five days alone at their current camp. Her friends would pick her up on their way back.

Fortunately, Renee gradually improved. By the time her friends returned, she was able to make the several-day struggle back to the cars. It was a trip Renee likely will never forget. And although Renee didn't have many positive things to say about those ten days, she was forcibly impressed with at least one thing: a single dietary indiscretion can cause days of pain.

As sad as that story of a backpacking trip gone awry is, it pales into insignificance when compared to the heartbreaking account of Sam Ballard.[299] At the age of 19, Sam was a strapping Australian rugby player. One day while relaxing with his friends, they spied a garden slug on the patio. Sam swallowed it on a dare.

Over the next days to weeks Sam's health deteriorated. He was ultimately diagnosed with rat lungworm infection caused by the microbe, *Angiostrongylus cantonensis*. The parasite then invaded his brain, causing something called eosinophilic meningoencephalitis.[300] That was only the beginning of his ordeal. Sam fell into a coma for some 420 days. He finally awoke a quadriplegic, confined to a wheelchair. Eight years later at the age of 28 he died.

Sam Ballard's story, like Renee's, reminds us that we should be very circumspect when it comes to the things we ingest. Granted, these are relatively unusual stories. Most of us are guilty of dietary indiscretions on a regular basis, yet don't end up victims in a horror story. However, accounts like those involving Renee and Sam are sobering because they remind us that what we ingest can have serious and sometimes unexpected consequences.

It is possible that you would never think of eating food that even had the slightest taste of spoilage. It's also likely you will never pick up a garden pest and eat it for dessert. But are you carelessly ingesting other things that should also generate serious concerns?

One Place Where Our Guard is Often Down: The Dietary Supplements Aisle

When it comes to dietary supplements, herbs, and other natural products, I've noticed that many people let down their guard. Even though there is typically little regulatory oversight of these supplements, millions of people down such foreign substances because they saw a compelling internet video, or because Aunt Nellie said it helped her, or because a neighbor shared a story of some medical miracle.

Years ago, Sherry came to our residential health center with a diagnosis of rheumatoid arthritis. She had packed in her luggage some bags of a "Chinese herb" purported to cure arthritis. During the course of her stay, she made remarkable progress. We wondered how much of her improvement might be due to the Chinese herbal supplement. Despite our best efforts we couldn't find someone who could give us an accurate translation of the exclusively Chinese writing on the packages. A couple of weeks later, we learned that even the best Chinese translator wouldn't have helped us. The herbal supplement did not contain its purported constituents. An FDA report revealed that the "natural" supplement, known as *Chuifong Toukuwan*, was filled with powerful drugs including pain killers, diuretics, and tranquilizers. Yes, Sherry felt better, but it was not because of the power of herbs—she was taking powerful prescription drugs, posing as "herbal supplements."[301]

The story of the FDA's analysis does not end there, however. Although the supplements were illicitly laden with drugs calculated to help a variety of symptoms, they were also contaminated with heavy metals like lead and cadmium.

This latter point is especially worth highlighting. Many supplements over the years have been found to be tainted by metals[302] which, you may have guessed, can wreak havoc on your Methuselah Factor and circulatory health.[303]

This point was graphically illustrated in my own clinical practice some years ago when Waldo came in with neurological complaints. Our evaluation uncovered arsenic poisoning. Some subsequent detective work by the public health department and a university toxicologist uncovered the source: a multi-vitamin and mineral supplement that Waldo was taking to improve his health.

OK, you say. I've convinced you to stay away from rotten food, slugs, and foreign supplements whose ingredient lists you can't read. However, the concerns with agents purporting to be natural far transcend the scenarios we've looked at. Consider the case of another heavy metal. This time our focus shifts to iron.

When I was a boy, iron had all the luster of gold. I can remember commercials touting iron as the ideal pick-me-up for individuals struggling with fatigue. Even today, many doctors routinely put pregnant women on iron, increasing its reputation for safety and health enhancement.

However, we don't have to go further than the obstetrics literature to realize that something is wrong with the common iron narrative. Simply put, although supplementing with iron is very important for the iron deficient, ingesting more of this mineral may be more dangerous than beneficial for many others. At the heart of the concerns is this: Iron in excess acts as a pro-oxidant. It thus carries the potential to ramp up inflammatory processes in our bodies, and with that to undermine our Methuselah Factor.

Although ongoing debate exists in the medical research literature, a number of studies suggest that giving iron routinely to any segment of the population may be particularly dangerous, especially for individuals who already have adequate iron stores.[304] For example, give every pregnant woman iron-containing supplements and a number of studies indicate you put them at greater risk for pregnancy-related diabetes and high blood pressure (preeclampsia and eclampsia).[305]

More Supplements of Concern

A host of herbs and supplements can stimulate our sympathetic nervous systems, putting us at risk for high blood pressure, elevated stress hormone levels, and worsened blood fluidity. Among those supplements are a number that we highlighted in our book, *Thirty Days to Natural Blood Pressure Control.* Here are some of the herbs and supplements that are best avoided if you want to optimize your Methuselah Factor, your blood pressure, and your metabolism:[306,307,308]

- 1,3-dimethylamylamine (1,3-DMAA)
- 1,3-dimethylbutylamine (1,3-DMBA)
- 1,4-dimethylamylamine (1,4-DMAA)
- 2-amino-6-methylheptane (octodrine)
- Arnica (*Arnica montana*)

- Beta-methylphenylethylamine (BMPEA)

- Bitter orange (*Citrus aurantium*)

- Ephedra or Ma Huang (*Ephedra sinica*)

- Ginkgo (*Ginkgo bilboa*)

- Ginseng (*Panax quinquefolias* and *Panax ginseng*)

- Guarana (*Paullinia cupana*)

- Higenamine (norcoclaurine or demethylcoclaurine)

- Kava (*Piper methysticum*)

- Kola nut (*Cola nitida* and *Cola acuminata*)

- Licorice (*Glycyrrhiza glabra*)

- Methylsynephrine (oxilofrine)

- Senna (*Cassia senna*)

- St. John's wort (*Hypericum perforatum*)

- Yohimbine (*Pausinystalia yohimbe*)

It is worth noting that the list above contains stimulants that have been banned in the U.S. like 1,3-dimethylamylamine (1,3-DMAA) and 1,3-dimethylbutylamine (1,3-DMBA). Nonetheless, these ingredients continue to be used in supplements sold in the States.[309]

If you haven't already picked up on it, here's my main message from today's chapter: If you are taking any supplements that have not been prescribed by your doctor, or adopted based on specific counsel in this book or elsewhere (like a vitamin D supplement or magnesium), then I want you to consider stopping them for the remainder of the program.

If you are an ardent supplement adherent, don't despair, in our next chapter I'll highlight additional supplements or herbal therapies that might be worth your attention. And for those of you who just want to wash your hands of the whole subject, I won't compel you tomorrow to take a supplement that you don't need. After all, there's no question: lifestyle is the optimal approach for boosting your Methuselah Factor, not popping some natural pills.

And, one other thing: if this chapter has you thinking more about avoiding food contaminants, leaving off those expensive supplements will give you a little more cash to select more certified organic produce that can further decrease your toxin exposures.

41

DAY 27: BEFRIEND
SOME BIOLOGICALS

Today's Challenge: Consider adding a medically-validated, Methuselah-Factor-enhancing supplement to your daily regimen.

FOR FIVE YEARS A 28-year-old African woman, who I'll call Armelle, had been afflicted with progressive neurological complications. She was plagued by burning sensations on her back and upper chest, numbness and tingling in her arms and legs, and foot and hand weakness. In addition, Armelle suffered from insomnia and irritability. Over those five years Armelle was seen by "numerous health institutions for which she had been treated for diverse pathologies," but experienced no abating of her symptoms. This neurologically-challenged young woman was finally evaluated by health professionals at the Grace Community Health and Development Association in Kumba, Cameroon (West Africa). There Armelle was diagnosed with vitamin B_{12} deficiency. Because injectable B_{12} was not readily available in Kumba, she was treated with high dose oral supplementation (2000 mcg daily). After only one month of such treatment, Armelle's symptoms improved dramatically.[310]

Although the authors of the scientific paper relating Armelle's story indicated that vitamin B_{12} deficiency is apparently rarely seen in young patients in Cameroon, worldwide the condition is extremely common. The likelihood of manifesting vitamin B_{12} deficiency is greatly increased by advancing age and the use of medications like metformin (used commonly for diabetes) and omeprazole and related *prazole* drugs (used for gastrointestinal conditions like heartburn and ulcers). Armelle herself had been on omeprazole (sold in the U.S. under the brand name, Prilosec) for a number of years.

To further illustrate how widespread is vitamin B_{12} deficiency, consider some other data. In a South African study of 121 patients (average age of 58.5) who were taking metformin for diabetes, 28.1% of them were vitamin B_{12} deficient. Among 60 Bhutanese refugees (from Nepal) living in Minnesota, 32% of them tested positive for B_{12} deficiency.[311] In large studies in the U.S. and the U.K. about 6% of the population over 60 years of age are B_{12} deficient using fairly strict criteria (< 148 pmol/L).[312] Many more individuals may be suffering from vitamin B_{12} lack who do not have such profoundly low levels.

I've opened this chapter with a focus on vitamin B_{12} for several reasons. First as we've observed, it is much more common than many people (even health professionals) realize. Second, it is extremely treatable, particularly if caught before serious irreversible complications occur. Third, if you haven't already guessed, the medical research literature suggests that B_{12} deficiency may be linked to poorer hemorheology. For example, deficiency of this vitamin has been linked to more rigid red blood cells that are more likely to clump together.[313]

So, after asking you to get rid of all your supplements in the last chapter, I'm now going to address several supplements that you should be taking, or at least consider taking. One of those supplements is vitamin B_{12}. Because supplementation is simple and quite inexpensive, I generally recommend everyone take in the range of 500 micrograms daily. If you're in your 20s or 30s, you can probably get away with as little as 50 micrograms per day. However, if you're in your 60s or older you're probably better off with 1000-2000 micrograms per day (the latter figure is the amount recommended for those with B_{12} absorption problems). Previous research has suggested that vitamin B_{12} is best absorbed if you take a supplement that contains only B_{12} (i.e., not a multivitamin supplement) and that you chew it, take it under your tongue, or allow it to otherwise dissolve in your mouth.[314]

Throughout this book, I've been making a case for eating as close as possible to a whole foods, plant-based diet. However, if you're not yet eating a particularly plant-strong diet, there may be some other supplements worth considering.

Ranking high among other dietary constituents that improve blood fluidity are the omega-3 fats. These polyunsaturated fats help deliver far-reaching benefits, including a decreased risk of heart problems, lower levels of a harmful blood fat known as triglycerides, and better blood pressure, not to mention favorable effects on hemorheology.[315] For example, omega-3 fats make platelets less likely to clump, thus improving one's Methuselah Factor.[316]

If you are regularly eating items like ground flax, chia seeds, or walnuts, you may well be getting plenty of omega-3 fats. However, over the years, it has seemed like the diets of most of my patients could have been improved by adding some additional omega-3 sources.

At this point, a word of caution is warranted. If you remember my concerns in the last chapter regarding heavy metals and their adverse effects on hemorheology, you'll likely want to steer away from fish as your primary source of omega-3 fats. Fish are among the most toxin-laden foods on the planet, exposing us to chemicals that can further worsen the Methuselah Factor. For example, mercury contamination of seafood offsets some of the cardiovascular benefits of omega-3 fats.[317,318] Furthermore, no fish on planet earth make omega-3 fats; they are only made by plants. Some fish do concentrate the omega-3 fats in their tissues, however, when they eat various ocean "plants" like phytoplankton.[319]

If, despite my advice, you choose to get your omega-3 fats from fish or fish oil, common recommendations are that you consume in the range of *5000 mg per week* of the *long chain* omega-3 fats found in those sources. In contrast, the omega-3 fats in plants (alpha linolenic acid or ALA) are referred to as *short-chain* fats although they only have 2 to 4 less carbons in their fatty-acid chains (18 carbons vs 20 or 22 carbons). In other words, the long-chain and the short-chain fats are quite similar in length. Since our bodies can convert ALA to the longer chain fats with some difficulty, I recommend more liberal intake of the plant sources to some patients, so that they will be taking *up to 15,000 mg per day.* Consider data adapted from a graphic in our book, *Thirty Days to Natural Blood Pressure Control*, to provide an idea of natural ways to work up to that much omega-3 fat intake.[320] Approximately 1000 - 1250 mg of ALA is found in:

- 1/2 teaspoon of flaxseed oil
- 1/4 ounce of chia seeds
- 1/3 cup of walnuts
- 2 teaspoons of ground flax

However, omega-3 supplementation is not for everyone,

especially in higher dosages. Special caution is warranted if you are on blood thinning medications or drugs that require critical blood levels like those used to treat HIV or prevent organ rejection.

Help for Iron Overload

In the previous chapter, I raised some concerns about excess iron and its potential to harm your Methuselah Factor. Some of you may have already translated that caution into action. If you hadn't already donated blood in the last four weeks, you may have made a beeline to the local blood bank and finally parted with some of that vital fluid. It's true: one way to decrease the iron load in your body is by donating blood. However, there appear to be other ways of offsetting the heart-harming and/or hemorheology-impairing effects of heavy metals like iron, lead, and mercury. One viable strategy is taking a zinc supplement.

On one hand, chronic zinc deficiency is associated with a host of problems including poorer immune function and worsened inflammation.[321] On the other hand, adequate body zinc levels can play a role in countering the oxidative stress imposed by other heavy metals.[322] This has been illustrated in a population group that we looked at closely in the previous chapter, pregnant women. Excess iron was associated with potentially deleterious effects during pregnancy, while zinc generally appears to play a protective role.[323]

With zinc, you can get too much of a good thing. In general, I recommend limiting elemental zinc intake from supplements to no more than 25 mg per day.

Beware of the Newest Methuselah Factor Supplement

As the Methuselah Factor becomes more popular in lay circles, I expect enterprising supplement purveyors to promote a host of plant products that "improve hemorheology." The research indicates that there are hundreds of plants that may possess such properties.[324] However, some of these plants will not have a long-term track record of safety. In fact, if the past is any guide, supplement marketers will tend to focus on less commonly known, or available, plant products. The reasons for this appear to relate both to the perception of novelty as well as the difficulty that consumers will have gaining access to alternative sources. Consequently on the grounds of safety and cost, I recommend only using novel biologicals to treat specific conditions that medical research supports, not on preventive grounds to improve blood fluidity.

However, there are a host of dietary plants that have been consumed for centuries with a solid track record of safety. Many of them have chemical constituents that hold promise for improving the Methuselah Factor.[325] I would encourage you to get the most cutting-edge mix of these emerging hemorheology enhancers—not by buying a supplement off the shelf, but rather by boosting your intake of plant products.

So, you have a relatively simple assignment before you today. Take a close look at vitamin B_{12}, omega-3 fats and zinc. Consider if one or more of them might not be an asset to your Methuselah-Factor-focused program. If so, add those supplements to your daily regimen as you enter the home stretch of our thirty-day journey.

42

DAY 28: FORGIVE

Today's Challenge: Extend forgiveness to at least one person who has wronged you—and you have not already forgiven. (Optional: perform at least one act of unmerited kindness each day.)

SEVEN YEARS AGO, Dr. Buck Blodgett seemed to have it all. Buck had a successful chiropractic practice in a Midwestern community. He was esteemed and loved by many inside and outside his practice. He had a strong and stable family, living with his loving wife and devoted teen-aged daughter.

However, all that changed in a matter of hours. Buck's beloved daughter, Jessie, his only child, was brutally raped and murdered, in her own bedroom by an intruder.

How do you deal with the unthinkable? As Dr. Blodgett records in his book, *A Message from Jessie*, he quickly realized how he needed to respond to the gruesome murder: with forgiveness.[326]

We've all heard the forgiveness narratives before. When

I reflect on those stories, they seem to invariably spring from strong faith traditions: the Amish families in Lancaster County, Pennsylvania, grieving over the mass murder of their daughters;[327] the Holocaust survivors who fall back on their religious roots;[328] those traumatized by the murders in Charleston, South Carolina's Emanuel African Methodist Episcopal Church.[329] However, there was a notable difference when it came to Buck Blodgett: he was a self-proclaimed atheist.

After the release of his book, I had the privilege of interviewing Dr. Blodgett on my weekly radio show.[330] His on-air reflections were both fascinating and provocative. Consider the following: "I know for me how life-changing and profound and powerful it [forgiveness] has been... I just feel blessed in a crazy way, I feel like had we [my wife and I] not had that forgiveness from the beginning, we would have taken an entirely different path the last three and a half years, and it would not have been good, and wouldn't have felt good, and it wouldn't have turned out well."

When discussing the *how* of forgiveness Buck reflected, "I feel like forgiveness is from a higher place. I feel like it came to me and through me, not from me."

As I thought about that interview, Dr. Buck Blodgett forcibly reminded me and my listeners that forgiveness is not in the exclusive domain of the religious. Regardless of our faith backgrounds, forgiveness can be employed to help heal ourselves and our world.

All of this is extremely relevant as we look at optimizing our Methuselah Factor. After all, we have noted throughout this book that one effective way of undermining your hemorheology is by ramping up your stress hormones. When wronged, we can respond in stress-enhancing ways, like harboring anger and hostility,[331] or we can exercise mercy and forgiveness. We have already noted how anger and hostility tend to worsen blood fluidity.[332] Expressing anger can be particularly destructive to the Methuselah Factor.

For example, Swiss researchers found that worry, anger, and hostility all tended to raise levels of clotting Factor VII,[333] which is linked to poor hemorheology.[334] On the other side of the Atlantic, researchers from the University of Pittsburg, using nationwide data, found that anger expression was linked to levels of the inflammatory compound, interleukin 6 (IL-6), as well as the hemorheology-undermining clotting factor, fibrinogen.[335] Furthermore, their data pointed to racial differences that raised concerns about how the effects of historical trauma, discrimination, and mistreatment might impact one's response to being wronged.

In short, the same research that reveals linkages between anger, hostility, and poor blood fluidity presents evidence for avoiding judgmentalism. I should see my being wronged as a call for me to forgive; but should not rush to judgment as to why someone else is not more forgiving.

Furthermore, forgiveness provides the foundation for healing broken relationships—and rebuilding trust. Depending on the intensity of the wrong, trust can take days or even years to be rebuilt. Nonetheless, forgiveness sets the foundation upon which such rebuilding can occur. When looked at from the standpoint of hemorheology, trusting relationships are extremely important. By way of contrast, when cynical distrust exists, inflammation rises and hemorheology worsens, as attested to by worsening levels of IL-6, C-reactive protein, and fibrinogen.[336]

The Challenge to Forgive

As we are winding up our thirty-day program, today's challenge is to identify someone who has wronged you and to offer them forgiveness. Although this is one of the most difficult tasks to address emotionally, it may be one of the most powerful aspects of our one-month journey. There's a benefit to presenting this element late in the program: you're either going to follow my advice and accept this challenge (even if your actual interaction with the person who harmed you takes place shortly after our thirty-day program concludes) or you will feel this is simply too difficult a request. In the latter scenario, you won't have this challenge facing you for more than another couple of days.

Steps to Forgiveness

Psychologists have offered a number of strategies to help us more effectively forgive. One helpful construct was offered by Drs. Stefanie and Elisha Goldstein.[337] The material that follows was inspired and informed by their insights. It was complemented by Tom Valeo's observations in a WebMD article entitled "Forgive and Forget."[338]

1. **Acknowledge your pain.** We often overlook opportunities for forgiveness because we have buried our pain and hurt. Sometimes that suppressed pain is due to blaming ourselves, excusing the guilt of a wrongdoer *because we feel that we didn't measure up*. The reality is this: no one has a right to treat you with disrespect or unkindness—no matter what you have done. Allow yourself to feel the pain that has come at the hand of the one who wronged you.

2. **Don't misunderstand forgiveness.** Forgiveness does not mean you condone the wrong done you. Instead, you are releasing the wrong doer from any "right" you have to take revenge. As the Goldsteins put it, you make "the conscious choice to release yourself from the burden, pain, and stress of holding on to resentment." Valeo quotes Charlotte vanOyen Witvliet, PhD, to address another mistaken aspect of forgiveness: "Forgiveness does not involve a literal

forgetting. Forgiveness involves remembering graciously. The forgiver remembers the true though painful parts, but without the embellishment of angry adjectives and adverbs that stir up contempt."

3. **Change your narrative.** Don't tell yourself and others that you are a victim, but rather re-imagine yourself as a survivor, overcoming adverse life experiences. Share that narrative with yourself and others. Tom Valeo turned to another expert to clarify this important point. Frederic Luskin, PhD, Director of the Stanford University Forgiveness Projects, went on record, "You can change, 'I hate my mother because she didn't love me,' to, 'Life is a real challenge for me because I didn't feel loved as a child.' That makes forgiveness so much more possible."

4. **Walk in the perpetrator's shoes.** When we are victimized it can be hard to see any positive qualities in the one who wronged us. However, the medical literature reveals that those who abuse others were often once abused themselves. Again, none of this excuses destructive behavior. Nonetheless, trying to see through the perpetrator's eyes can help us cultivate compassion. This is extremely important because when someone wrongs us they actually entrust us with incredible power. Really. We can blame them, shame them, or seek revenge. On the other hand, we can offer them undeserved forgiveness. If they accept this gift, it can provide the grounds upon which to rebuild their life and relationships.

5. **Reflect on the blessings of forgiveness.** Think of a time when you did something wrong and someone extended forgiveness to you. Gratefully reliving that experience can help you cultivate a more gracious posture.

6. **Recognize the two facets of forgiveness.** In an earlier work, my co-authors and I put it this way: "Full forgiveness is a two-way street, where the one wronged first chooses to forgive, and then the wrongdoer actually accepts that forgiveness. Genuine acceptance of forgiveness occurs only when the perpetrator recognizes and admits to his wrongdoing and repents."[339] In other words, you first choose to forgive on a decisional level. You make "a conscious, deliberate decision to release feelings of resentment or vengeance toward a person or group who has harmed you, regardless of whether they actually deserve your forgiveness."[340] However, the second aspect to forgiveness involves actually confronting the perpetrator and letting him or her know that you have forgiven them. Depending on the nature of the wrongdoing and the personality of the wrongdoer, it may not be safe to do this in person. In some cases, law enforcement may need to be informed of the act(s) of victimization so that the perpetrator can be separated from you or other potential victims. Taking legal recourse does not mean you are unforgiving. Recognizing that someone is dangerous to themselves or others may call for extreme measures. However, even in these situations you can still offer forgiveness.

7. **Remember, you're not alone.** If you find it difficult to forgive or confront the perpetrator (or if you have concerns about whether or not confrontation is safe at present), then get help. Although sharing concerns with a close friend or spiritual leader might be beneficial, having the support of a mental health professional is often invaluable. Don't be afraid to get that professional help.

8. **Strive for emotional forgiveness.** It is true that forgiveness at its heart involves a choice where we step away from

angry and vengeful thoughts directed at the perpetrator. Psychologists refer to this as *decisional forgiveness*. However, a significant time can pass before a person moves from such a decision into what is called *emotional forgiveness*. When you experience emotional forgiveness, you will harbor thoughts like love, compassion, and empathy toward the wrongdoer rather than feelings of resentment, bitterness, and anger. This should be our ultimate goal. However, to reiterate, it can take time, sometimes lots of time.

9. **Be patient.** Even though I'm giving you this assignment toward the end of our program, it doesn't mean that forgiveness will necessarily come easily. Many psychologists view forgiveness as a process rather than as a simple act. If you can think of a number of ways in which you've been wronged, why not begin by extending forgiveness to someone for a smaller transgression?

10. **See forgiveness as a pathway to strength and growth.** It's easy to focus on the difficulty of forgiving and say, "Why do I need to do this anyway?" It's true, receiving forgiveness can be transformational for the perpetrator; however, it can also be life-changing for you when you extend it— even if it is difficult. Just as our physical muscles get stronger by stressing ourselves in a weight room, so our emotional "muscles" strengthen when dealing with the stress of those who have wronged us. As the Goldsteins expressed it: "As you practice working with the pain that's there, you grow key strengths of self-compassion, courage, and empathy that inevitably make you stronger in every way... even in the most horrific and painful circumstances, we have the freedom to create meaning in life, which is a powerful healing agent."

An Alternative Challenge: Cultivate Kindness

If you feel that asking you to forgive is too much to tackle at this point (or if you can't think of a single person in the world who you haven't forgiven), I have an additional challenge in this chapter: perform at least one act of *unmerited kindness* each day for the rest of the program. This alternative challenge is actually related to forgiveness. Think about it: forgiveness is an extreme act of unmerited, and even undeserved, kindness. On the other hand, alerting a stranger who is about to pull out of the grocery store's parking lot to an item she left on the lower rack of her shopping cart would be a more simple, and probably not an overwhelming, act of unmerited kindness. In contrast, offering your neighbor some tomatoes from your garden may or may not qualify as unmerited. If your neighbor never did anything nice for you, it would clearly be unmerited. If, on the other hand, that same neighbor had just yesterday brought you some cucumbers from his garden, it would appear that you performed an act of *merited* kindness (some could say you felt obligated to share based on his past kindness toward you).

How do you know if a kind act is merited or unmerited? Usually if you perform it for a stranger, it's unmerited. When the recipient is a close friend or family member, honestly ask yourself whether or not you have any social obligation to do the "kindness." If your answer is *yes*, then that particular activity might still be very good to do, but it doesn't allow you to check off today's assignment.

As you probably guessed, there's a scientific basis for challenging you to practice deeds of kindness. Kind acts have been linked to psychological well-being.[341] This in turn, has been shown to make us more likely to engage in health enhancing behaviors,[342] as well as offering benefits to our blood fluidity in and of itself.[343]

Kindness Ideas

Unmerited acts of kindness are sometimes called *random acts of kindness*. Others use the *random* designation only with *unplanned* acts. Definitions aside, there are a number of organizations that exist to promote kindness. Two of them are the *Random Acts of Kindness Foundation* and *Random Acts*. Looking for some ideas on how to fulfill today's challenge? Figure 22 offers some ideas that I've either taken directly, or adapted, from their pages.[344,345] I've employed a construct used by *Random Acts* where the time commitments involved in the activities are indicated.

You have your challenge for today that will continue into the two days remaining in our program. Why not plan right now to do something kind for someone who doesn't deserve it? And, if you really want to be bold, think of someone whom you need to forgive—and start moving in that direction.

FIGURE 22	Examples of Unmerited Acts of Kindness

Time Commitment	Examples of Acts of Kindness
Less Than a Minute	– Compliment someone for their good qualities – Leave quarters at the laundromat – Even when provoked, be polite on the road – Leave a generous tip – Give away your parking spot – Let someone go ahead of you in line – Pay for someone in line behind you
Several Minutes to an Hour	– Start a fundraiser for a worthy cause – Write a positive sticky note to brighten up someone's day – Send an encouraging postcard, letter, or text – Write a positive comment on a website or blog – Gift an inspirational book

FIGURE 22 (CONTINUED)	Examples of Unmerited Acts of Kindness

Time Commitment	Examples of Acts of Kindness
A Few Hours	– Donate blood – Help a physically-challenged friend or neighbor with household chores – Bake some bread for your local fire or police station
One to Several Days	– Have a "judgment-free" day when you say nothing critical about anything or anyone – Organize an event to clean up a public park, roadway, or other public space – Volunteer for a day at a shelter
A Few Weeks	– Organize a food drive for the needy – Help coordinate a blood drive – Organize a book drive for your library
One Month or More	– Start or support a community garden – Mentor at-risk youth – Provide free help in an area where you have expertise

43

DAY 29: MAKE FRIENDS WITH MELATONIN

Today's Challenge: Plan to boost melatonin's effects on your body—either by following lifestyle practices to increase melatonin production or by taking a controlled-release melatonin supplement.

YEARS AGO, MY CHILDREN became enamored with melatonin during an intercontinental plane trip. Several families were traveling with us, sharing a common goal of doing some charitable work overseas. As you might have guessed, during that long flight, our collective children, who ranged in age from about 7 to 14, negotiated with their parents to ensure they could all sit in close proximity. Everything went well for several hours until, as I later learned, some of the kids got tired of the antics of a child I'll call Ralph. Without any parental input, some of the children duped Ralph into downing one or two melatonin pills (they passed them off as candy). As the story was later related to me, about thirty minutes after his melatonin "treat," Ralph fell asleep, and remained in "dream land" for the remainder of that extended flight.

Whether or not melatonin had anything to do with Ralph's somnolence, the medical research is convincing when it comes to melatonin's sleep-enhancing properties.[346] However, this natural compound has emerged as far more than a sleep aid. Melatonin also has been documented to help with blood pressure lowering,[347,348] a variety of liver and intestinal diseases and conditions,[349,350] cancer prevention,[351,352] immune system enhancement,[353] and a number of other conditions (including the effects of aging) that are related to oxidation.[354] Furthermore, melatonin appears to provide anxiety relief and other benefits to children with autism spectrum disorder.[355]

Because the benefits of melatonin seem to overlap those of the Methuselah Factor, we shouldn't find it surprising if melatonin directly improved blood fluidity. Indeed, research has linked melatonin to enhanced hemorheology.[356] For example, researchers from Switzerland demonstrated that a single dose of only 3 mg of melatonin causes measurable decreases in two important blood clotting proteins, Factor VIII:C and fibrinogen.[357] In addition, melatonin supplementation may offer additional Methuselah Factor benefits if we are facing a variety of significant stressors.[358,359]

Of the different formulations of melatonin, the controlled-release variety appears to be the most efficacious, at least when it comes to blood pressure lowering.[360,361] A typical dosage used in blood pressure studies is 2 to 3 mg of *controlled-release, or slow release*, melatonin per night. However, if taking a fast-release preparation, such levels of supplementation may be excessive. Richard Wurtman, MD, is an internationally renowned brain chemistry researcher who currently holds the position of Cecil H. Green Distinguished Professor, Department of Brain and Cognitive Sciences, at the Massachusetts Institute of Technology.

Dr. Wurtman recommends taking no more than 0.3 to 0.5 mg of the fast-release melatonin nightly.[362] In contrast to the story of Ralph, which opened this chapter, research suggests that melatonin may be most effective in inducing sleep if it is taken two hours before bedtime.[363,364]

For today's challenge I want you to do one of two things: either start taking a bedtime melatonin supplement or review your lifestyle practices to optimize your body's own production of melatonin. That's right, we can boost our melatonin levels without relying on supplementation. Melatonin is produced by the pineal gland, a small structure that is housed within the brain. Lifestyle factors can either enhance or impair melatonin production.

In addition, we now know that melatonin can also be made by the cells lining our intestinal tract.[365] Lifestyle factors also can influence intestinal melatonin production. Foremost among these appears to be the avoidance of evening snacks, ensuring you go to bed with an empty stomach, and declining blood sugar levels.[366] Finally, melatonin can also be found in certain plant sources of nutrition.

With our thirty-day journey nearly complete, the supplement option may sound more attractive than further lifestyle changes do. Although supplementation generally appears to be safe, there are at least two major concerns with taking melatonin supplements. First, if melatonin is obtained from the brains of animals, some have expressed theoretical concerns about transmissible brain infections. Second, in the more likely scenario of synthetic melatonin use, the pills are often tainted with byproducts of the chemical production process. A recent review identified 13 contaminants or classes of contaminants found in melatonin supplements.[367] Some have definite or potential human toxicity. Among the former is 1,1'-ethylidenebis-(tryptophan), the infamous "peak E" that caused an incurable muscle disease known as

Eosinophilia-Myalgia Syndrome (EMS). Other melatonin supplement contaminants include:

- 1,2,3,4-tetrahydro-β-carboline-3-carboxylic acid
- 3-(phenylamino)alanine
- 2-(3-indolylmethyl)-tryptophan
- formaldehyde-melatonin
- formaldehyde-melatonin condensation products
- 5-methoxy-tryptamine derivatives
- N-acetyl- and diacetyl-indole derivatives
- 1,3-diphthalimidopropane
- hydroxy-bromo-propylphthalimide
- chloropropylphthalimide

Although melatonin supplementation has a good track record and is generally safe[368] (in part, because contaminants occur in very tiny amounts), long term use of anything, especially when it contains known contaminants, should at least cause us to consider other options. When Neil Nedley, MD, wrote his popular book, *Proof Positive: How to Reliably Combat Disease and Achieve Optimal Health Through Nutrition and Lifestyle*, he advocated using lifestyle strategies to raise melatonin levels.[369] His review of the evidence has been underscored and extended by subsequent authors on the topic.[370] Why not choose to ensure you are following the melatonin-boosting practices in Figure 23? After all, most of them are already familiar as elements of *The Methuselah Factor Diet and Lifestyle Program*.

Go for it. Embrace, or recommit to, as many of the lifestyle factors in Figure 23 as you can reasonably surround. If that's too difficult a challenge, then consider taking a melatonin supplement on a nightly basis.

FIGURE 23	Natural Strategies to Boost Melatonin

Category	Examples or Other Details
Go to bed early	On or before 10 PM appears to be optimal
Before bedtime, avoid portable light-emitting devices	Tablets, smartphones, etc.
Sleep in total darkness	Use a blindfold or eye mask, if necessary
During daylight hours, get bright light exposure	Outdoor sunshine or the equivalent
Avoid non-prescription drugs known, or suspected, to suppress melatonin production	– Caffeine – Alcohol – Tobacco – Sleep aids – Nonsteroidal Anti-inflammatory drugs
Talk with your prescriber about working to limit use of other medications that may adversely affect melatonin levels	– Antianxiety agents – Antidepressents – Sleeping pills – Certain blood pressure pills such as beta and calcium channel blockers

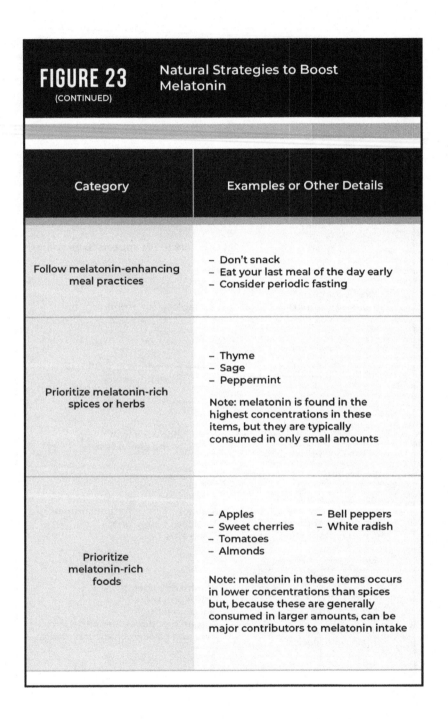

Category	Examples or Other Details
FIGURE 23 (CONTINUED)	**Natural Strategies to Boost Melatonin**
Follow melatonin-enhancing meal practices	– Don't snack – Eat your last meal of the day early – Consider periodic fasting
Prioritize melatonin-rich spices or herbs	– Thyme – Sage – Peppermint Note: melatonin is found in the highest concentrations in these items, but they are typically consumed in only small amounts
Prioritize melatonin-rich foods	– Apples – Bell peppers – Sweet cherries – White radish – Tomatoes – Almonds Note: melatonin in these items occurs in lower concentrations than spices but, because these are generally consumed in larger amounts, can be major contributors to melatonin intake

44

DAY 30: SIGN UP FOR
A MARATHON

Today's Challenge: Commit to sticking with at least one of your new lifestyle habits for an additional thirty days. Consider hosting a "Methuselah Factor" or natural blood pressure program for your community.

DURING AN INTERVIEW ON my syndicated radio show, orthopedic surgeon, Edgar O. Vyhmeister, MD, shared a remarkable story. He related how a gentleman, who we'll call Robert, sought orthopedic care for severe hip arthritis. Appropriately, plans were made for total hip replacement surgery.

However, on the day of surgery, things went terribly wrong. Before the orthopedist could begin the procedure, Robert had a heart attack while undergoing anesthesia. He was quickly awakened, and given the bad news. The surgery was cancelled, and Robert found himself in the Coronary Care Unit rather than the recovery room.

The sudden change of events motivated Robert to do all he could to optimize his heart health. Robert learned of the heart benefits of "a plant-based" diet, an approach to eating shown to help reverse the very blockages in coronary arteries that cause heart attacks.[371] In short order, Robert adopted such an eating strategy. Although Robert likely never heard of "the Methuselah Factor" or "hemorheology," he was making lifestyle changes that were calculated to dramatically improve his blood fluidity.

After six months, his orthopedist told Robert, "I think you're now ready to have your total hip replacement." However, Robert had a surprising response: "My hip is feeling better. I don't think I want a total hip replacement." Dr. Vyhmeister later had an opportunity to review Robert's X-rays. He saw something remarkable. The original films, taken shortly before his heart attack, showed severe "bone-on-bone" arthritis. After his months on a Methuselah-Factor-optimizing lifestyle, Robert's X-rays had improved significantly. Vyhmeister saw evidence of cartilage regeneration.

During our interview, Dr. Vyhmeister was careful to point out that he didn't expect this to be healthy normal joint cartilage, but rather an alternate form of cushioning tissue known as *fibrocartilage*. Nonetheless, this regenerated tissue was having a profound effect in lessening Robert's pain. To Dr. Vyhmeister's knowledge that improvement was so marked that Robert never required hip replacement.

If the take-home lesson is not already apparent, Dr. Vyhmeister removed any doubt for my radio listeners: these improvements occurred as a result of better circulation. This was not an isolated instance. Edgar went on to explain how since that time, he has shared this message with other orthopedic patients with similar results.

As remarkable as that story is, one detail bears special emphasis: Robert's improvements occurred over *six months*, not thirty days. In other words, had Robert been following *The Methuselah*

Factor Diet and Lifestyle Program as spelled out in the pages of this book, even on this concluding day of the journey, he may not have realized his most cherished goals.

In contrast to Robert's six-month-long healing journey, consider results from three different community programs that used our *Thirty Days to Natural Blood Pressure Control* book and related DVDs to host a "Lowering High Blood Pressure Naturally" seminar.[372] Figure 24 shows the pooled results from 25 men and women with high blood pressure (defined, for our analysis, as a systolic blood pressure of greater than, or equal to, 140 mmHg).

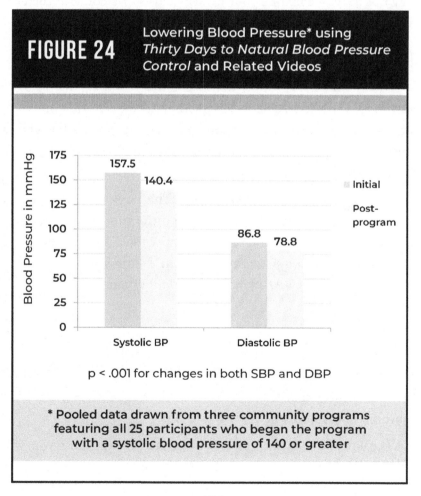

FIGURE 24 — Lowering Blood Pressure* using *Thirty Days to Natural Blood Pressure Control* and Related Videos

p < .001 for changes in both SBP and DBP

*Pooled data drawn from three community programs featuring all 25 participants who began the program with a systolic blood pressure of 140 or greater

The programs depicted in Figure 24 were conducted over as short as thirty days and as long as eight weeks. The lifestyle and supplements promoted in the book and videos were such that significant improvements in the Methuselah Factor could be expected. However, in contrast to Robert's six-month-long process, the average participant logged remarkable improvements *in as little as thirty days*. This included a 17-point drop in systolic blood pressure—without adding additional medications!

I share these two scenarios to make an important point: as powerful as *The Methuselah Factor Diet and Lifestyle* is, you may or may not have reached all your health goals as we come to the conclusion of our thirty-day journey.

Sign Up for a Marathon

It is with that background that I challenge you to *sign up for a marathon*. I realize such a charge may immediately conjure up ideas of competitive athletics. And although there may be value in preparing for a physical endurance race, I'm talking about something altogether different.

We made a deal at the beginning of this book that we would go on a thirty-day journey together. When the sun sets today, you're done with your side of the bargain. You worked hard, scrutinizing your lifestyle for ways to improve your Methuselah Factor. You made changes and saw benefits. No doubt, you faced challenges along the way.

However, now you are at an important juncture. Where do you go from here? You are not obligated to continue any of the lifestyle factors that you embraced during the past month. However, I would suggest that there are two categories of responses as you continue to map out the rest of your life.

The first type of response is illustrated by those of you who have made tremendous progress during the past thirty days. You might reasonably respond: "I'd be a fool to not continue this entire program for the rest of my life." I realize those may sound like strong words. However, it's merely a paraphrase of Hector, a patient I told you about in Chapter 14.

If you are wondering about more of the context, Hector had signed up for a two-week residential lifestyle change program. At the conclusion of the program, he admitted he initially had no intention of following the lifestyle that he had embarked on a couple weeks earlier. However, when he evaluated his progress (including pre- and post-program lab work), he shared with a group of participants what was on his heart, "I'd be a fool to not continue this entire program for the rest of my life."

I'm hopeful that you, like Hector, checked your blood work at the beginning of this program and will reevaluate it in the next few days, if you've not done so already. I'm optimistic that you've been keeping track of some of your other measurements and recording them in Figure 16. If you have been monitoring your progress, there's a good chance that you're like Hector. You have made so much improvement that you just want to continue this new lifestyle indefinitely.

The second type of response is heard from those who might feel like Robert in our opening illustration. Although we don't know how he felt thirty days into his six-month regimen, it is possible he hadn't yet noticed any remarkable changes. Or to make it even more tangible, you could be like a patient of ours named "Juan," whom we wrote about in *Thirty Days to Natural Blood Pressure Control*.

Juan came to the same residential program that Hector later attended. Juan's single focus was lowering his elevated triglycerides (a type of blood fat that is connected to multiple health risks).

After two weeks of serious lifestyle changes, Juan was both disappointed and angered when he received his end-of-program blood work. His triglycerides had actually increased!

Fortunately, Juan accepted his physician's counsel to not give in to his emotions, but rather to stick with the overall healthy lifestyle he had embraced. Six months later Juan's triglycerides had dropped dramatically. He was now a happy man with a firmly entrenched healthy lifestyle!

This second category of response could be articulated: "I've *not* made the progress that I wanted, but I believe in the program and will stick with it."

I realize that some of you may not fall into either of the two extremes which I've mentioned. It is very possible that you made some improvement but have not fully reached your goals. You may be excited about some progress, but disappointed by other areas where you have not seen the changes that you hoped for. So, regardless of where you fall on that great continuum, here's my message: Lifestyle change is much more like a marathon than a sprint. And even though the past thirty days may have seemed like an endurance race, one month is just a sprint from the perspective of the rest of our lives.

So, here is today's challenge: sign up for a marathon. Look at all you've changed over the past month and make a serious decision about what will be different going forward. You may want to continue to follow all the program elements you embraced. You may opt to stick with only some of them. But don't jettison the entire program. If you haven't seen the progress that you have hoped for, that's all the more reason to try to continue to follow things carefully—at least for another month.

Help for the Journey

Most serious athletes that I have known over the years were part of a team. This was true even if they competed in an individual sport, like marathon running. It is likely they were part of a track team or an athletic club. They may have had a running partner or partners and a coach who made "the journey" with them. Similarly, as you prepare to run your lifestyle marathon for at least the next month (and, ideally, the rest of your life), it really helps to be part of a team.

Before I provide some suggestions, let me address concerns that may be percolating in your semiconscious mind (if you've not already expressed them out loud). Some of you might be comparing this chapter to the classic *bait and switch* or the act of *upselling* you on a product that you never wanted. After all, I asked you to sign on to *The Methuselah Factor Diet and Lifestyle Program* only for thirty days. Now I'm talking with you about thirty more days—and even the rest of your life!

Look, we all have to make lifestyle choices every day—and that will continue until we close our eyes in that last final sleep. I'm challenging you to apply what you learned over the last thirty days, and I'm making the case that, if your results were not what you expected, then you should be just as diligent as the person who made stunning progress.

With all this in mind, let me tell you now about resources for building a team to help you on your journey from here on out. I already introduced you to those resources, in Chapter 19, when we talked about connecting with others. Specifically, we have free on-line videos and inexpensive DVDs that can help you build a supportive community. In a moment, I'll review those resources with you. But, for now, I want to reiterate—and expand—my challenge. I want you to sign up for a marathon. Look at all the lifestyle changes that you have made over the past thirty days and commit to continuing at least some of them for the next month. To increase your likelihood of success, I want you to strongly consider finding a "running partner" who is going to train alongside you for the next thirty days. Let me frame it this way: I want you to commit to *helping someone else* succeed on this program over *the next thirty days*.

When you partner with someone else, it will both increase their likelihood of success—and help to solidify your personal gains from the program. Now here's four possible ways to help you do it:

1. **Develop your own program.** You and one or more friends can choose to read this book together. Of course, this doesn't mean you have to sit down in the same room for a reading session. The idea is that you're reading or re-reading (in your case) this book on the same schedule. Granted, you may just be scanning the chapters as they read them for the first time. Maybe you'll pick up the audiobook edition and listen to me read to you during your morning commute. You get the idea.

   But developing your own program also involves some structured interaction. Maybe you will join up with a healthy lifestyle group in your community. Perhaps you will work out together at a local health club. Maybe you'll opt for a group walk or bike ride on a regular basis. The idea is to craft your own program, one that meets your needs.

2. **Use our free on-line videos.** If you have not already been using my daily YouTube videos, they provide a great resource to support those who join you on your next thirty-day journey. The best launching place for those videos is www.compasshealth.net/diabetes-bp. I recommend that

each participant watch the daily videos in addition to going through this book. Plan some time, at least weekly, to share your experience and insights together—even if that meeting must take place by phone.

Remember that although the video series is entitled *30 Days to Natural Diabetes and High Blood Pressure Control*, my filmed remarks take you over similar ground as that covered in Chapters 15 to 44 of this book. The only major difference is that the videos focus strictly on diabetes and high blood pressure rather than on the broader theme of hemorheology.

3. **Host a weekly** *Methuselah Factor Diet and Lifestyle Program* in your home, workplace, local library, or faith community center. With the help of two inexpensive DVD resources that feature my instructional and motivational messages, you can lead a once-weekly seminar or support group that meets five times over a thirty-day span. This same program is sometimes offered under the name, *Thirty Days to Abundant Health*. Regardless of the name you choose to use for your seminar, the delivery of the program is flexible. It can be as simple as encouraging participants to read this book daily, meeting once a week to watch a video, and then asking for feedback. You can find full details at www.compasshealth.net/the-methuselah-factor.

4. **Host a** *Lowering Your Blood Pressure Naturally* **program** in your home or other public or private venue. This program is ideal if you have neighbors, coworkers, or family members who are more interested in a program that targets a specific medical condition like high blood pressure, rather than a comprehensive health series like *The Methuselah Factor Diet and Lifestyle Program*. Our blood

pressure program involves eight sessions that are delivered over the course of four to eight weeks (twice weekly for four weeks, or once per week for eight weeks). You can find full details at www.compasshealth.net/hypertension. This series centers on our book, *Thirty Days to Natural Blood Pressure Control*, and related DVD materials. Because it covers a similar range of lifestyle topics, you can also use this book and the free on-line videos (www.compasshealth. net/diabetes-bp/) to complement the material.

You've got plenty of options for the future. You don't have to train for, or run in, life's marathon on your own. Make a commitment to continue selected elements of *The Methuselah Factor Diet and Lifestyle Program* for the next thirty days, and make sure you bring someone else along for the journey.

45

PARTING WORDS

CONGRATULATIONS. YOU HAVE TAKEN major strides to improve not only your own health but the health of your family, your community, and our planet. I know that may seem like hyperbole, but it's not. Over the past thirty days we've seen how improving our blood fluidity can positively impact health in dramatic ways.

Reflect seriously on where you've come from and take the challenge of Chapter 44. Find some way to reinforce the program in your own life and, then, share it with others. You will be thankful that you did.

ENDNOTES

1. Weimar Institute. NEWSTART program. www.newstart.com. Accessed 22 November 2018.

2. Wildwood Lifestyle Center. www.wildwoodhealth.org. Accessed 22 November 2018.

3. See, for example:

   European Society for Microcirculation. National Societies. http://www. esmicrocirculation.eu/nationalsocieties.html. Accessed 22 November 2018.

   The British Microcirculation Society. http://www.microcirculation.org.uk/. Accessed 22 November 2018.

   Union of International Associations. International Society for Clinical Haemorheology (ISCH). *Open Yearbook*. 2018. Accessed 22 November 2018.

   The International Society of Biorheology. http://www.coe.ou.edu/isb/. Accessed 22 November 2018.

   The European Society for Clinical Hemorheology and Microcirculation http://www3.unisi.it/ricerca/asso/esch/index.htm. Accessed 22 November 2018.

4. Merriam-Webster.com. Hemorheology. https://www.merriam-webster.com/ medical/hemorheology. Accessed 22 November 2018.

5. White EG. *Healthful Living*. 1898. Fort Oglethorpe, GA: TEACH Services, Inc., p. 30.

6. Szapary L, Horvath B, et al. Hemorheological disturbances in patients with chronic cerebrovascular diseases. *Clin Hemorheol Microcirc*. 2004;31(1):1-9.

7. Ibid.

8. See, for example: McKay F. A history on the use of blood transfusions in cycling. Parts 1-3. *Cycling News*. February 27 – March 7, 2013.

9. Joyner MJ. VO2MAX, blood doping, and erythropoietin. *Br J Sports Med.* 2003 Jun;37(3):190-1.

10. Gerrard DF. Playing foreign policy games: States, drugs and other Olympian vices. *Sport in Society.* 2008; 11(4):459-466.

11. Allport LE, Parsons MW, et al. Elevated hematocrit is associated with reduced reperfusion and tissue survival in acute stroke. *Neurology.* 2005 Nov 8;65(9):1382-7.

12. Sandhagen B. Red cell fluidity in hypertension. *Clin Hemorheol Microcirc.* 1999;21(3-4):179-81.

13. Sakuta S. Blood filterability in cerebrovascular disorders, with special reference to erythrocyte deformability and ATP content. *Stroke.* 1981 Nov-Dec;12(6):824-8.

14. Berker M, Dikmenoglu N, et al. Hemorheology, melatonin and pinealectomy. What's the relationship? An experimental study. *Clin Hemorheol Microcirc.* 2004;30(1):47-52.

15. Cho YI, Cho DJ. Hemorheology and microvascular disorders. *Korean Circ J.* 2011 Jun;41(6):287-95.

16. Yarnell JW, Baker IA, et al. Fibrinogen, viscosity, and white blood cell count are major risk factors for ischemic heart disease. The Caerphilly and Speedwell collaborative heart disease studies. *Circulation.* 1991 Mar;83(3):836-44.

17. Yarnell JW, Patterson CC, et al. Haemostatic/inflammatory markers predict 10-year risk of IHD at least as well as lipids: the Caerphilly collaborative studies. *Eur Heart J.* 2004 Jun;25(12):1049-56.

18. Cecchi E, Liotta AA, et al. Relationship between blood viscosity and infarct size in patients with ST-segment elevation myocardial infarction undergoing primary percutaneous coronary intervention. *Int J Cardiol.* 2009 May 15;134(2):189-94.

19. Peters SA, Woodward M, et al. Plasma and blood viscosity in the prediction of cardiovascular disease and mortality in the Scottish Heart Health Extended Cohort Study. *Eur J Prev Cardiol.* 2017 Jan;24(2):161-167.

20. Cohen MC, Rohtla KM, et al. Meta-analysis of the morning excess of acute myocardial infarction and sudden cardiac death. *Am J Cardiol.* 1997; 79:1512.

21. Kimura T, Inamizu T, et al Determinants of the daily rhythm of blood fluidity. *J Circadian Rhythms.* 2009 Jun 26;7:7.

22. Koenig W, Ernst E. The possible role of hemorheology in atherothrombo-genesis. *Atherosclerosis.* 1992 Jun;94(2-3):93-107.

23. Wikipedia contributors. Kirby Puckett. *Wikipedia, The Free Encyclopedia.* https://en.wikipedia.org/w/index.php?title=Kirby_Puckett&oldid=867893273. Updated 8 November 2018. Accessed 22 November 2018.

24. Trope GE, Salinas RG, Glynn M. Blood viscosity in primary open-angle glaucoma. *Can J Ophthalmol.* 1987 Jun;22(4):202-4.

25. Wu ZJ, Li MY. Blood viscosity and related factors in patients with primary open-angle glaucoma [translated abstract]. *Zhonghua Yan Ke Za Zhi.* 1993 Nov;29(6):353-5.

26. See, for example: Kilic-Toprak E, Toprak I, et al. Increased erythrocyte aggregation in patients with primary open angle glaucoma. *Clin Exp Optom.* 2016 Nov;99(6):544-549.

27. Lip PL, Blann AD, et al. Age-related macular degeneration is associated with increased vascular endothelial growth factor, hemorheology and endothelial dysfunction. *Ophthalmology.* 2001 Apr;108(4):705-10.

28. von Tempelhoff GF, Nieman F, et al. Association between blood rheology, thrombosis and cancer survival in patients with gynecologic malignancy. *Clin Hemorheol Microcirc.* 2000;22(2):107-30.

29. Seebacher V, Polterauer S, et al. The prognostic value of plasma fibrinogen levels in patients with endometrial cancer: a multi-centre trial. *Br J Cancer.* 2010 Mar 16;102(6):952-6.

30. Jain S, Harris J, Ware J. Platelets: linking hemostasis and cancer. *Arterioscler Thromb Vasc Biol.* 2010 Dec;30(12):2362-7.

31. Vona G, Sabile A, et al. Isolation by size of epithelial tumor cells: a new method for the immunomorphological and molecular characterization of circulating tumor cells. *Am J Pathol.* 2000 Jan;156(1):57-63.

32. Jain S, Harris J, Ware J. Op. cit.

33. Gorudko IV, Shamova EV, et al. Glutathione-dependent regulation of platelet aggregation with neutrophils and tumor cells [English abstract]. *Biofizika.* 2012 Jan-Feb;57(1):93-8.

34. Elwood PC, Pickering J, Gallacher JEJ. Cognitive function and blood rheology: results from the Caerphilly cohort of older men. *Age and Ageing.* 2001 Vol: 30(2):135-139.

35. Ibid.

36. Chang CY, Liang HJ, et al. Hemorheological mechanisms in Alzheimer's disease. *Microcirculation.* 2007 Aug;14(6):627-34.

37. Cicco G, Cicco S. The influence of oxygen supply, hemorheology and microcirculation in the heart and vascular systems. *Adv Exp Med Biol.* 2010;662:33-9.

38. Cicco G, Pirrelli A. Red blood cell (RBC) deformability, RBC aggregability and tissue oxygenation in hypertension. *Clin Hemorheol Microcirc.* 1999;21(3-4):169-77.

39. Sugimori H, Tomoda F, et al. Blood rheology and platelet function in untreated early-stage essential hypertensives complicated with metabolic syndrome. *Int J Hypertens.* 2012;2012:109830.

40. Kamhieh-Milz S, Kamhieh-Milz J, et al. Regular blood donation may help in the management of hypertension: an observational study on 292 blood donors. *Transfusion.* 2016 Mar;56(3):637-44.

41. American Diabetes Association. Statistics About Diabetes. http://www.diabetes.org/diabetes-basics/statistics/. Updated 22 March 2018. Accessed 22 November 2018.

42. World Health Organization. *Global Report on Diabetes.* 2016. Geneva, Switzerland: WHO Press, p. 6.

43. Ibid.

44. Although clinicians will sometimes talk about Type 1B diabetes, Type 1.5 diabetes, or other designations, for practical purposes, dividing all diabetes into Type 1 and Type 2 is probably the most practical.

45. Johnson JL, Duick DS, et al. Identifying prediabetes using fasting insulin levels. *Endocr Pract.* 2010 Jan-Feb;16(1):47-52.

46. Koltai K, Feher G, et al. The effect of blood glucose levels on hemorheological parameters, platelet activation and aggregation in oral glucose tolerance tests. *Clin Hemorheol Microcirc.* 2006;35(4):517-25.

47. Brun JF, Aloulou I, Varlet-Marie E. Hemorheological aspects of the metabolic syndrome: markers of insulin resistance, obesity or hyperinsulinemia? *Clin Hemorheol Microcirc.* 2004;30(3-4):203-9.

48. Meigs JB, Mittleman MA, et al. Hyperinsulinemia, hyperglycemia, and impaired hemostasis: the Framingham Offspring Study. *JAMA.* 2000 Jan 12;283(2):221-8.

49. Sugimori H, Tomoda F, et al. Blood rheology and platelet function in untreated early-stage essential hypertensives complicated with metabolic syndrome. *Int J Hypertens.* 2012;2012:109830.

50. Nakanishi N, Yoshida H, et al. White blood-cell count and the risk of impaired fasting glucose or type II diabetes in middle-aged Japanese men. *Diabetologia.* 2002;45(1):42-48.

51. Luft VC, Schmidt MI, et al. Chronic inflammation role in the obesity-diabetes association: a case-cohort study. *Diabetol Metab Syndr.* 2013 Jun 27;5(1):31.

52. Serné EH, Meijer RI, et al. Microvascular dysfunction: Potential role in the pathogenesis of obesity-associated hypertension and insulin resistance (Chapter 4). In: Wiernsperger N, Bouskela E, Kraemer-Aguiar LG, eds. *Microcirculation and Insulin Resistance.* 2009. Bentham Science Publishers Ltd., p. 41-54.

53. See, for example:

    Barbieri M, Ragno E, et al. New aspects of the insulin resistance syndrome: impact on haematological parameters. *Diabetologia.* 2001 Oct;44(10):1232-7.

    Choi KM, Lee J, et al. Relation between insulin resistance and hematological parameters in elderly Koreans-Southwest Seoul (SWS) Study. *Diabetes Res Clin Pract.* 2003 Jun;60(3):205-12.

    Ellinger VC, Carlini LT, et al. Relation between insulin resistance and hematological parameters in a Brazilian sample. *Arq Bras Endocrinol Metabol.* 2006 Feb;50(1):114-7.

    Hanley AJ, Retnakaran R, et al. Association of hematological parameters with insulin resistance and beta-cell dysfunction in nondiabetic subjects. *J Clin Endocrinol Metab.* 2009 Oct;94(10):3824-32.

54. Oltmanns KM, Gehring H, et al. Hypoxia causes glucose intolerance in humans. *Am J Respir Crit Care Med.* 2004 Jun 1;169(11):1231-7.

55. Siervo M, Riley HL, et al. Effects of prolonged exposure to hypobaric hypoxia on oxidative stress, inflammation and gluco-insular regulation: the not-so-sweet price for good regulation. *PLoS One.* 2014 Apr 14;9(4):e94915.

56. Serné EH, Meijer RI, et al. Op.cit.

57. Wong TY, Klein R, et al. Retinal arteriolar narrowing and risk of diabetes mellitus in middle-aged persons. *JAMA.* 2002 May 15;287(19):2528-33.

58. Cho YI, Mooney MP, Cho DJ. Hemorheological disorders in diabetes mellitus. *J Diabetes Sci Technol.* 2008 Nov;2(6):1130-8.

59. Koltai K, Feher G, et al. The effect of blood glucose levels on hemorheological parameters, platelet activation and aggregation in oral glucose tolerance tests. *Clin Hemorheol Microcirc.* 2006;35(4):517-25.

60. Millward D. Before and after: the transformation of US dieting industry. *The Telegraph.* https://www.telegraph.co.uk/business/2018/02/17/transformation-us-dieting-industry/. 17 February 2018. Accesssed 8 May 2018.

61. U.S. Centers for Disease Control and Prevention (CDC). Overweight and obesity. https://www.cdc.gov/obesity/data/adult.html. Updated 13 August 2018. Accessed 23 November 2018.

62. For example, see: Barnes JN, Nualnim N, et al. Macro- and microvascular function in habitually exercising systemic lupus erythematosus patients. *Scand J Rheumatol.* 2014;43(3):209-16.

63. For example, see: Santos MJ, Pedro LM, et al. Hemorheological parameters are related to subclinical atherosclerosis in systemic lupus erythematosus and rheumatoid arthritis patients. *Atherosclerosis.* 2011 Dec;219(2):821-6.

64. For example, consider the following research on the autoimmune conditions of systemic sclerosis and scleroderma:

   Harris ES, Meiselman HJ, et al. Successful long-term (22 year) treatment of limited scleroderma using therapeutic plasma exchange: Is blood rheology the key? *Clin Hemorheol Microcirc.* 2017;65(2):131-136.

   Korsten P, Niewold TB, et al. Increased whole blood viscosity is associated with the presence of digital ulcers in systemic sclerosis: Results from a cross-sectional pilot study. *Autoimmune Dis.* 2017;3529214.

65. Blackwell DL, Lucas JW, Clarke TC. Summary health statistics for U.S. adults: National Health Interview Survey, 2012. National Center for Health Statistics. *Vital Health Stat* 10(260). 2014.

66. Kauppila LI. Atherosclerosis and disc degeneration/low-back pain--a systematic review. *Eur J Vasc Endovasc Surg.* 2009 Jun;37(6):661-70.

67. Ha IH, Lee J, et al. The association between the history of cardiovascular diseases and chronic low back pain in South Koreans: a cross-sectional study. *PLoS One.* 2014 Apr 21;9(4):e93671.

68. Antony B, Venn A, et al. Association of body composition and hormonal and inflammatory factors with tibial cartilage volume and sex difference in cartilage volume in young adults. *Arthritis Care Res* (Hoboken). 2016 Apr;68(4):517-25.

69. Teng ZY, Pei LC, et al. Whole blood viscosity is negatively associated with bone mineral density in postmenopausal women with osteoporosis. *Bone*. 2013 Oct;56(2):343-6.

70. Ye C, Xu M, et al. Decreased bone mineral density is an independent predictor for the development of atherosclerosis: a systematic review and meta-analysis. *PLoS One*. 2016 May 5;11(5):e0154740.

71. Yarnell JW, Fehily AM, et al. Determinants of plasma lipoproteins and coagulation factors in men from Caerphilly, South Wales. *J Epidemiol Community Health*. 1983 Jun;37(2):137-40.

72. Simmonds MJ, Meiselman HJ, Baskurt OK. Blood rheology and aging. *J Geriatr Cardiol*. 2013 Sep;10(3):291-301.

73. Kowal P, Hurla G. Age and hemorheologic changes in stroke. *Acta Clin Croat* 2000; 39:273-276.

74. Mohebali D, Kaplan D, et al. Alterations in platelet function during aging: clinical correlations with thromboinflammatory disease in older adults. *J Am Geriatr Soc*. 2014 Mar;62(3):529-35.

75. Kowal P, Hurla G. Op. cit.

76. Simmonds MJ, Meiselman HJ, Baskurt OK. Blood rheology and aging. *J Geriatr Cardiol*. 2013 Sep;10(3):291-301.

77. Ujiie H, Kawasaki M, et al. Influence of age and hematocrit on the coagulation of blood. *J Biorheology*. 2009 Dec;23(2):111-114.

78. Simmonds MJ, Meiselman HJ, Baskurt OK. Op. cit.

79. Cesari M, Kritchevsky SB, et al. Oxidative damage and platelet activation as new predictors of mobility disability and mortality in elders. *Antioxid Redox Signal*. 2006 Mar-Apr;8(3-4):609-19.

80. Kim JY, Kim OY, et al. Association of age-related changes in circulating intermediary lipid metabolites, inflammatory and oxidative stress markers, and arterial stiffness in middle-aged men. *Age (Dordr)*. 2013 Aug;35(4):1507-19.

81. Senturk UK, Yalcin O, et al. Effect of antioxidant vitamin treatment on the time course of hematological and hemorheological alterations after an exhausting exercise episode in human subjects. *J Appl Physiol* (1985). 2005 Apr;98(4):1272-9.

82. Lafay S, Jan C, et al. Grape extract improves antioxidant status and physical performance in elite male athletes. *J Sports Sci Med*. 2009 Sep 1;8(3):468-80.

83. Peternelj TT, Coombes JS. Antioxidant supplementation during exercise training: beneficial or detrimental? *Sports Med*. 2011 Dec 1;41(12):1043-69.

84. Myburgh KH. Polyphenol supplementation: benefits for exercise performance or oxidative stress? *Sports Med*. 2014 May;44 Suppl 1:S57-70.

85. Bouix D, Peyreigne C, et al. Relationships among body composition, hemorheology and exercise performance in rugbymen. *Clin Hemorheol Microcirc*. 1998 Nov;19(3):245-54.

86. Brun JF, Varlet-Marie E, et al. Blood rheology and body composition as determinants of exercise performance in female rugby players. *Clin Hemorheol Microcirc*. 2011;49(1-4):207-14.

87. See, for example: Késmárky G, Kenyeres P, et al. Plasma viscosity: a forgotten variable. *Clin Hemorheol Microcirc*. 2008;39(1-4):243-6.

88. Notice that the final column to the right in Figure 16 is labeled "Other Improvements." This gives you some flexibility to list personalized goals. Wondering about what else to measure? Recently, I've become interested in something called the PULS test. It gives a single score based on a variety of blood tests that have a bearing on hemorheology, inflammation, and other indicators of circulatory health. You can learn more at http://www.pulstest.com/ or by reviewing the following scientific paper: Cross DS, McCarty CA, et al. Coronary risk assessment among intermediate risk patients using a clinical and biomarker based algorithm developed and validated in two population cohorts. *Curr Med Res Opin*. 2012 Nov;28(11):1819-30.

89. Blais CA, Pangborn RM, et al. Effect of dietary sodium restriction on taste responses to sodium chloride: a longitudinal study. *Am J Clin Nutr*. 1986 Aug;44(2):232-43.

90. Gnasso A, Cacia M, et al. No effect on the short-term of a decrease in blood viscosity on insulin resistance. *Clin Hemorheol Microcirc*. 2018;68(1):45-50.

91. Kamhieh-Milz S, Kamhieh-Milz J, et al. Regular blood donation may help in the management of hypertension: an observational study on 292 blood donors. *Transfusion*. 2016 Mar;56(3):637-44.

92. Bani-Ahmad MA, Khabour OF, et al. The impact of multiple blood donations on the risk of cardiovascular diseases: Insight of lipid profile. *Transfus Clin Biol*. 2017 Nov;24(4):410-416.

93. Shin S, Ku YH, Ho JX, et al. Progressive impairment of erythrocyte deformability as indicator of microangiopathy in type 2 diabetes mellitus. *Clin Hemorheol Microcirc*. 2007;36(3):253-61.

94. Adams RA, Higgins T, et al. The effect of physical activity on haemato-logical predictors of cardiovascular risk: evidence of a dose response. *Clin Hemorheol Microcirc*. 2012;52(1):57-65.

95. Adapted from the Physical Activity Readiness Questionnaire (PAR-Q).

96. Simpson HC, Simpson RW, et al. A high carbohydrate leguminous fibre diet improves all aspects of diabetic control. *Lancet*. 1981 Jan 3;1(8210):1-5.

97. Singhal P, Kaushik G, Mathur P. Antidiabetic potential of commonly con-sumed legumes: a review. *Crit Rev Food Sci Nutr*. 2014;54(5):655-72.

98. Suárez-Martíneza SE, Ferriz-Martíneza RA, et al. Bean seeds: leading nutraceutical source for human health (review). *CyTA – Journal of Food*. 2016;14(1):131–137.

99. Zia-Ul-Haq M, Ahmed S, et al. Report: Platelet aggregation inhibi-tion activity of selected legumes of Pakistan. *Pak J Pharm Sci*. 2012 Oct;25(4):863-5.

100. Zia-ul-Haq M, Khan BA, et al. Platelet aggregation and anti-inflamma-tory effects of garden pea, Desi chickpea and Kabuli chickpea. *Acta Pol Pharm*. 2012 Jul-Aug;69(4):707-11.

101. Wirtz PH, Redwine LS, et al. Independent association between lower level of social support and higher coagulation activity before and after acute psychosocial stress. *Psychosom Med*. 2009 Jan;71(1):30-7.

102. Maughan RJ, Griffin J. Caffeine ingestion and fluid balance: a review. *J Hum Nutr Diet*. 2003 Dec;16(6):411-20.

103. Chou T. Wake up and smell the coffee. Caffeine, coffee, and the medical consequences. *West J Med*. 1992 Nov;157(5):544-53.

104. Giardina E. Cardiovascular effects of caffeine and caffeinated beverages. *UpToDate*. Updated 19 October 2017. Accessed 23 November 2018.

105. Chou T. Op. cit.

106. Loftfield E, Shiels MS, et al. Associations of coffee drinking with systemic immune and inflammatory markers. *Cancer Epidemiol Biomarkers Prev.* 2015 Jul;24(7):1052-60.

107. Cornelis MC, El-Sohemy A, et al. Coffee, CYP1A2 genotype, and risk of myocardial infarction. *JAMA.* 2006 Mar 8;295(10):1135-41.

108. Xie Y, Qin J, et al. Coffee consumption and the risk of lung cancer: an updated meta-analysis of epidemiological studies. *Eur J Clin Nutr.* 2016 Feb;70(2):199-206.

109. Zeng SB, Weng H, et al. Long-term coffee consumption and risk of gastric cancer: A PRISMA-compliant dose-response meta-analysis of prospective cohort studies. *Medicine (Baltimore).* 2015 Sep;94(38):e1640.

110. Sinha R, Cross AJ, et al. Caffeinated and decaffeinated coffee and tea intakes and risk of colorectal cancer in a large prospective study. *Am J Clin Nutr.* 2012 Aug;96(2):374-81.

111. Caini S, Cattaruzza MS, et al. Coffee, tea and caffeine intake and the risk of non-melanoma skin cancer: a review of the literature and meta-analysis. *Eur J Nutr.* 2017 Feb;56(1):1-12.

112. DeRose DJ, Braman MA, et al. Alternative and complementary therapies for nicotine addiction [abstract]. *Complementary Health Practice Review* 2000 Fall; 6(1):98.

113. Freedman ND, Park Y, et al. Association of coffee drinking with total and cause-specific mortality. *N Engl J Med.* 2012 May 17;366(20):1891-904.

114. Sagon C. Want to live longer? Drink coffee. *Healthy Living* (AARP Blog). http://blog.aarp.org/2012/05/17/want-to-live-longer-drink-coffee/. Posted 17 May 2012. Accessed 29 June 2018.

115. Anson J, Anson O. Death rests a while: holy day and Sabbath effects on Jewish mortality in Israel. *Soc Sci Med.* 2001 Jan;52(1):83-97.

116. Jews who observe the biblical principles spelled out in the Torah (the first five books of the Judeo-Christian Old Testament) keep a weekly Sabbath from sundown Friday to sundown Saturday. See, for example, Exodus 20:8-11 and Leviticus 23:32.

117. See, for example: Levi F, Halberg F. Circaseptan (about-7-day) bioperiodicity--spontaneous and reactive--and the search for pacemakers. *Ric Clin Lab.* 1982 Apr-Jun;12(2):323-70.

118. Mikulecky M Sr, Mikulecky M Jr. The Derer´s biological - cosmic week and the Halberg´s circaseptan chronome. *Bratisl Lek Listy.* 2014;115(4):243-6.

119. Reinberg AE, Dejardin L, et al. Seven-day human biological rhythms: An expedition in search of their origin, synchronization, functional advantage, adaptive value and clinical relevance. *Chronobiol Int.* 2017;34(2):162-191.

120. Haus E. Chronobiology of hemostasis and inferences for the chronotherapy of coagulation disorders and thrombosis prevention. *Adv Drug Deliv Rev.* 2007 Aug 31;59(9-10):966-84.

121. See, for example: Boivin DB, Boudreau P. Impacts of shift work on sleep and circadian rhythms. *Pathol Biol* (Paris). 2014 Oct;62(5):292-301.

122. Gan Y, Yang C, et al. Shift work and diabetes mellitus: a meta-analysis of observational studies. *Occup Environ Med.* 2015 Jan;72(1):72-8.

123. Vyas MV, Garg AX, et al. Shift work and vascular events: systematic review and meta-analysis. *BMJ.* 2012 Jul 26;345:e4800.

124. Abu Farha R, Alefishat E. Shift Work and the Risk of Cardiovascular Diseases and Metabolic Syndrome Among Jordanian Employees. *Oman Med J.* 2018 May;33(3):235-242.

125. Wang D, Ruan W, et al. Shift work and risk of cardiovascular disease morbidity and mortality: A dose-response meta-analysis of cohort studies. *Eur J Prev Cardiol.* 2018 Aug;25(12):1293-13021302.

126. Mattes RD. The taste for salt in humans. *Am J Clin Nutr.* 1997 Feb;65(2 Suppl):692S-697S.

127. Blais CA, Pangborn RM, et al. Effect of dietary sodium restriction on taste responses to sodium chloride: a longitudinal study. *Am J Clin Nutr.* 1986 Aug;44(2):232-43.

128. DeRose D, Steinke G, Li T. *Thirty Days to Natural Blood Pressure Control: The "No Pressure" Solution.* 2016. Foresthill, CA: CompassHealth Consulting Press, p. 104-114.

129. Azak A, Huddam B, et al. Salt intake is associated with inflammation in chronic heart failure. *Int Cardiovasc Res J.* 2014 Sep;8(3):89-93.

130. Yilmaz R, Akoglu H, et al. Dietary salt intake is related to inflammation and albuminuria in primary hypertensive patients. *Eur J Clin Nutr.* 2012 Nov;66(11):1214-8.

131. Liu F, Mu J, et al. Potassium supplement ameliorates salt-induced haemostatic abnormalities in normotensive subjects. *Acta Cardiol.* 2011 Oct;66(5):635-9.

132. Cornelissen VA, Fagard RH, et al. Impact of resistance training on blood pressure and other cardiovascular risk factors: a meta-analysis of randomized, controlled trials. *Hypertension*. 2011 Nov;58(5):950-8.

133. Garg R, Malhotra V, et al. Effect of isometric handgrip exercise training on resting blood pressure in normal healthy adults. *J Clin Diagn Res*. 2014 Sep;8(9):BC08-1010.

134. Farah BQ, Germano-Soares AH, et al. Acute and chronic effects of isometric handgrip exercise on cardiovascular variables in hypertensive patients: A systematic review. *Sports (Basel)*. 2017 Aug 1;5(3):55.

135. Baross AW, Hodgson DA, et al. Reductions in resting blood pressure in young adults when isometric exercise is performed whilst walking. *J Sports Med (Hindawi Publ Corp)*. 2017;2017:7123834.

136. Peters PG, Alessio HM, et al. Short-term isometric exercise reduces systolic blood pressure in hypertensive adults: possible role of reactive oxygen species. *Int J Cardiol*. 2006 Jun 16;110(2):199-205.

137. See, for example: Bizjak DA, Jacko D, et al. Acute alterations in the hematological and hemorheological profile induced by resistance training and possible implication for microvascular functionality. *Microvasc Res*. 2018 Jul;118:137-143.

138. American College of Sports Medicine. American College of Sports Medicine position stand. Progression models in resistance training for healthy adults. *Med Sci Sports Exerc*. 2009 Mar;41(3):687-708.

139. Fisher J, Steele J, et al. Evidence-based resistance training recommendations. *Medicina Sportiva* 2011 Sept;15(3): 147-162.

140. Signorile JF. Resistance training for older adults: Targeting muscular strength, power, and endurance. *ACSM's Health & Fitness Journal*. 2013 Sept/Oct;17(5):24-32.

141. Fisher J, Steele J, et al. Op. cit.

142. See, for example: Vessby B, Uusitupa M, et al. Substituting dietary saturated for monounsaturated fat impairs insulin sensitivity in healthy men and women: The KANWU Study. *Diabetologia*. 2001 Mar;44(3):312-9.

143. For the connection between diet and the delivery of amino acids needed by the brain to make serotonin (i.e., tryptophan) and dopamine (i.e., tyrosine), see: Wurtman RJ, Wurtman JJ, et al. Effects of normal meals rich in carbohydrates or proteins on plasma tryptophan and tyrosine ratios. *Am J Clin Nutr*. 2003 Jan;77(1):128-32.

144. James S, Vorster HH, et al. Nutritional status influences plasma fibrinogen concentration: evidence from the THUSA survey. *Thromb Res.* 2000 Jun 1;98(5):383-94.

145. Sanchez C, Poggi M, et al. Diet modulates endogenous thrombin generation, a biological estimate of thrombosis risk, independently of the metabolic status. *Arterioscler Thromb Vasc Biol.* 2012 Oct;32(10):2394-404.

146. Kimura S, Tamayama M, et al. Docosahexaenoic acid inhibits blood viscosity in stroke-prone spontaneously hypertensive rats. *Res Commun Mol Pathol Pharmacol.* 1998 Jun;100(3):351-61.

147. Rillaerts E, Van Camp K, et al. Blood viscosity parameters in coronary heart disease: effect of fish oil supplementation. *Acta Clin Belg.* 1989;44(1):17-23.

148. Connor WE. Importance of n-3 fatty acids in health and disease. *Am J Clin Nutr* 2000 Jan;71(1 Suppl):171S-5S.

149. Salonen JT, Nyyssönen K, et al. High stored iron levels are associated with excess risk of myocardial infarction in eastern Finnish men. *Circulation.* 1992 Sep;86(3):803-11.

150. Holay MP, Choudhary AA, Suryawanshi SD. Serum ferritin-a novel risk factor in acute myocardial infarction. *Indian Heart J.* 2012 Mar-Apr;64(2):173-7.

151. Rayman MP, Barlis J, et al. Abnormal iron parameters in the pregnancy syndrome preeclampsia. *Am J Obstet Gynecol.* 2002 Aug;187(2):412-8.

152. Siddiqui IA, Jaleel A, et al. Iron status parameters in preeclamptic women. *Arch Gynecol Obstet.* 2011 Sep;284(3):587-91.

153. See, for example:

Liu JL, Fan YG, et al. Iron and Alzheimer's disease: From pathogenesis to therapeutic implications. *Front Neurosci.* 2018 Sep 10;12:632.

Belaidi AA, Bush AI. Iron neurochemistry in Alzheimer's disease and Parkinson's disease: targets for therapeutics. *J Neurochem.* 2016 Oct;139 Suppl 1:179-197.

Dwyer BE, Zacharski LR, et al. Getting the iron out: phlebotomy for Alzheimer's disease? *Med Hypotheses.* 2009 May;72(5):504-9.

154. Mullington JM, Simpson NS, et al. Sleep Loss and Inflammation. *Best Pract Res Clin Endocrinol Metab.* 2010;24(5):775-784.

155. See, for example:

Koren D, Dumin M, Gozal D. Role of sleep quality in the metabolic syndrome. *Diabetes Metab* Syndr *Obes.* 2016 Aug 25;9:281-310.

Van Cauter E. Sleep disturbances and insulin resistance. *Diabet Med.* 2011 Dec;28(12):1455-62.

156. DeRose D, Steinke G, Li T. *Thirty Days to Natural Blood Pressure Control: The "No Pressure" Solution.* 2016. Foresthill, CA: CompassHealth Consulting Press, p. 182-184.

157. Cho YI, Cho DJ. Hemorheology and microvascular disorders. *Korean Circ J.* 2011 Jun;41(6):287-95.

158. Tripette J, Loko G, et al. Effects of hydration and dehydration on blood rheology in sickle cell trait carriers during exercise. *Am J Physiol Heart Circ Physiol.* 2010 Sep;299(3):H908-14.

159. Chan J, Knutsen SF, et al. Water, other fluids, and fatal coronary heart disease: the Adventist Health Study. *Am J Epidemiol.* 2002 May 1;155(9):827-33.

160. Mann JI, Appleby PN, et al. Dietary determinants of ischaemic heart disease in health conscious individuals. *Heart.* 1997 Nov;78(5):450-5.

161. Centers for Disease Control and Prevention (CDC). Fact Sheets - Alcohol Use and Your Health. https://www.cdc.gov/alcohol/fact-sheets/alcohol-use.htm. Updated 3 January 2018. Accessed 23 November 2018.

162. For example, see: Schütze M, Boeing H, et al. Alcohol attributable burden of incidence of cancer in eight European countries based on results from prospective cohort study. *BMJ.* 2011 Apr 7;342:d1584.

163. Choi SJ, Lee SI, Joo EY. Habitual alcohol consumption and metabolic syndrome in patients with sleep disordered breathing. *PLoS One.* 2016 Aug 18;11(8):e0161276.

164. Mayo Clinic Staff. Triglycerides: Why do they matter? https://www.mayoclinic.org/diseases-conditions/high-blood-cholesterol/in-depth/triglycerides/art-20048186?pg=2. Published 13 September 2018. Accessed 22 November 2018.

165. Cicha I, Suzuki Y, et al. Effects of dietary triglycerides on rheological properties of human red blood cells. *Clin Hemorheol Microcirc.* 2004;30(3,4):301–5.

166. Klop B, do Rego AT, Cabezas MC. Alcohol and plasma triglycerides. *Curr Opin Lipidol.* 2013 Aug;24(4):321-6.

167. GBD 2016 Alcohol Collaborators. Alcohol use and burden for 195 countries and territories, 1990-2016: a systematic analysis for the Global Burden of Disease Study 2016. *Lancet.* 2018 Sep 22;392(10152):1015-1035.

168. Ibid.

169. Solomon DH. Nonselective NSAIDs: Adverse cardiovascular effects. *UpToDate.* Updated 27 September 2017. Accessed 5 July 2018.

170. Ungprasert P, Srivali N, et al. Non-steroidal anti-inflammatory drugs and risk of venous thromboembolism: a systematic review and meta-analysis. *Rheumatology (Oxford).* 2015 Apr;54(4):736-42.

171. Snowden S, Nelson R. The effects of nonsteroidal anti-inflammatory drugs on blood pressure in hypertensive patients. *Cardiol Rev.* 2011 Jul-Aug;19(4):184-91.

172. DeRose D, Steinke G, Li T. Generic Names of Various Non-steroidal Anti-inflammatory Drugs, NSAIDS (Figure 13.1) in *Thirty Days to Natural Blood Pressure Control: The "No Pressure" Solution.* 2016. Foresthill, CA: CompassHealth Consulting Press, p. 281.

173. For example, see: Vogel VJ. *American Indian Medicine (The Civilization of the American Indian Series)*, Reprint edition. 1990. Oklahoma City, OK: The University of Oklahoma Press.

174. Iguchi M, Littmann AE, et al. Heat stress and cardiovascular, hormonal, and heat shock proteins in humans. *J Athl Train.* 2012 Mar-Apr;47(2):184-90.

175. Hussain J, Cohen M. Clinical effects of regular dry sauna bathing: A systematic review. *Evid Based Complement Alternat Med.* 2018 Apr 24;2018:1857413.

176. Wikipedia contributors. Spirituality. *Wikipedia, The Free Encyclopedia.* https://en.wikipedia.org/wiki/Spirituality. Updated 30 June 2018. Accessed 9 July 2018.

177. Herrera T. Why your brain tricks you into doing less important tasks. *New York Times* (online edition). https://www.nytimes.com/2018/07/09/smarter-living/eisenhower-box-productivity-tips.html. Published 9 July 2018. Accessed 22 November 2018.

178. Oken, BS. *Complementary Therapies in Neurology: An Evidence-Based Approach*. 2004. New York, NY: The Parthenon Publishing Group, p. 225.

179. Greenberg AS, Obin MS. Obesity and the role of adipose tissue in inflammation and metabolism. *Am J Clin Nutr*. 2006 Feb;83(2):461S-465S.

180. Hitsumoto T. Factors affecting impairment of blood rheology in obese subjects. *J Cardiol*. 2012 Nov;60(5):401-6.

181. Klöting N, Blüher M. Adipocyte dysfunction, inflammation and metabolic syndrome. *Rev Endocr Metab Disord*. 2014 Dec;15(4):277-87.

182. Wiewiora M, Piecuch J, et al. The impacts of super obesity versus morbid obesity on red blood cell aggregation and deformability among patients qualified for bariatric surgery. *Clin Hemorheol Microcirc*. 2014;58(4):543-50.

183. Church TS, Finley CE, et al. Relative associations of fitness and fatness to fibrinogen, white blood cell count, uric acid and metabolic syndrome. *Int J Obes Relat Metab Disord*. 2002 Jun;26(6):805-13.

184. Russo MA, Santarelli DM, O'Rourke D. The physiological effects of slow breathing in the healthy human. *Breathe (Sheff)*. 2017 Dec;13(4):298-309.

185. Byeon K, Choi JO, et al. The response of the vena cava to abdominal breathing. *J Altern Complement Med*. 2012 Feb;18(2):153-7.

186. Russo MA, Santarelli DM, O'Rourke D. Op. cit.

187. Lee JS, Lee MS, et al. Effects of diaphragmatic breathing on ambulatory blood pressure and heart rate. *Biomed Pharmacother*. 2003 Oct;57 Suppl 1:87s-91s.

188. Turin TC, Kita Y, et al. Ambient air pollutants and acute case-fatality of cerebro-cardiovascular events: Takashima Stroke and AMI Registry, Japan (1988-2004). *Cerebrovasc Dis*. 2012;34(2):130-9.

189. Bowe B, Xie Y, et al. The 2016 global and national burden of diabetes mellitus attributable to PM2·5 air pollution. *Lancet Planet Health*. 2018 Jul;2(7):e301-e312.

190. Czoli CD, Hammond D. TSNA Exposure: Levels of NNAL Among Canadian Tobacco Users. *Nicotine Tob Res*. 2015 Jul;17(7):825-30.

191. Higuchi T, Omata F, et al. Current cigarette smoking is a reversible cause of elevated white blood cell count: Cross-sectional and longitudinal studies. *Prev Med Rep*. 2016 Aug 9;4:417-22.

192. Ishizaka N, Ishizaka Y, et al. Relationship between smoking, white blood cell count and metabolic syndrome in Japanese women. *Diabetes Res Clin Pract.* 2007 Oct;78(1):72-6.

193. Belch JJ, McArdle BM, et al. The effects of acute smoking on platelet behaviour, fibrinolysis and haemorheology in habitual smokers. *Thromb Haemost.* 1984 Feb 28;51(1):6-8.

194. Ernst E. Haemorheological consequences of chronic cigarette smoking. *J Cardiovasc Risk.* 1995 Oct;2(5):435-9.

195. Bridges AB, Hill A, Belch JJ. Cigarette smoking increases white blood cell aggregation in whole blood. *J R Soc Med.* 1993 Mar;86(3):139-40.

196. See, for example: Salbaş K. Effect of acute smoking on red blood cell deformability in healthy young and elderly non-smokers, and effect of verapamil on age- and acute smoking-induced change in red blood cell deformability. *Scand J Clin Lab Invest.* 1994 Oct;54(6):411-6.

197. Anstey KJ, von Sanden C, et al. Smoking as a risk factor for dementia and cognitive decline: a meta-analysis of prospective studies. *Am J Epidemiol.* 2007 Aug 15;166(4):367-78.

198. Sabia S, Marmot M, et al. Smoking history and cognitive function in middle age from the Whitehall II study. *Arch Intern Med.* 2008 Jun 9;168(11):1165-73.

199. Wang X, Derakhshandeh R, et al. One minute of marijuana secondhand smoke exposure substantially impairs vascular endothelial function. *J Am Heart Assoc.* 2016 Jul 27;5(8).

200. Ghosh A, Basu D. Cannabis and psychopathology: The meandering journey of the last decade. *Indian J Psychiatry.* 2015 Apr-Jun;57(2):140-9.

201. Schmits E, Quertemont E. So called "soft" drugs: cannabis and the amotivational syndrome. [English abstract] *Rev Med Liege.* 2013 May-Jun;68(5-6):281-6.

202. Wang X, Derakhshandeh R, et al. Op. cit.

203. Holitzki H, Dowsett LE, et al. Health effects of exposure to second- and third-hand marijuana smoke: a systematic review. *CMAJ Open.* 2017 Nov 24;5(4):E814-E822.

204. Schuwald AM, Nöldner M, et al. Lavender oil-potent anxiolytic properties via modulating voltage dependent calcium channels. Skoulakis EMC, ed. *PLoS ONE.* 2013;8(4):e59998.

205. Sayorwan W, Siripornpanich V, et al. The effects of lavender oil inhalation on emotional states, autonomic nervous system, and brain electrical activity. *J Med Assoc Thai.* 2012 Apr;95(4):598-606.

206. DeRose D, Steinke G, Li T. *Thirty Days to Natural Blood Pressure Control: The "No Pressure" Solution.* 2016. Foresthill, CA: CompassHealth Consulting Press, p. 204-205.

207. Angelopoulos TJ, Lowndes J, et al. The effect of high-fructose corn syrup consumption on triglycerides and uric acid. *J Nutr.* 2009 Jun;139(6):1242S-1245S.

208. Cicha I, Suzuki Y, et al. Effects of dietary triglycerides on rheological properties of human red blood cells. *Clin Hemorheol Microcirc.* 2004;30(3,4):301–5.

209. Angelopoulos TJ, Lowndes J, et al. Op. cit.

210. Sloop GD, Bialczak JK, et al. Uric acid increases erythrocyte aggregation: Implications for cardiovascular disease. *Clin Hemorheol Microcirc.* 2016 Oct 5;63(4):349-359.

211. Malik VS, Schulze MB, Hu FB. Intake of sugar-sweetened beverages and weight gain: a systematic review. *Am J Clin Nutr* 2006 Aug;84(2):274-88.

212. Hammer MS, Swinburn TK, Neitzel RL. Environmental Noise Pollution in the United States: Developing an Effective Public Health Response. *Environmental Health Perspectives.* 2014;122(2):115-119.

213. Ibid.

214. Ibid.

215. Ndrepepa A, Twardella D. Relationship between noise annoyance from road traffic noise and cardiovascular diseases: a meta-analysis. *Noise Health.* 2011 May-Jun;13(52):251-9.

216. See, for example: Le Guen M, Nicolas-Robin A, et al. Earplugs and eye masks vs routine care prevent sleep impairment in post-anaesthesia care unit: a randomized study. *Br J Anaesth.* 2014 Jan;112(1):89-95.

217. Su TC, Hwang JJ, et al. Association between long-term exposure to traffic-related air pollution and inflammatory and thrombotic markers in middle-aged adults. *Epidemiology.* 2017 Oct;28 Suppl 1:S74-S81.

218. Lee H, Myung W, et al. Short- and long-term exposure to ambient air pollution and circulating biomarkers of inflammation in non-smokers: A hospital-based cohort study in South Korea. *Environ Int.* 2018 Oct;119:264-273.

219. Carey IM, Anderson HR, et al. Are noise and air pollution related to the incidence of dementia? A cohort study in London, England. *BMJ Open.* 2018 Sep 11;8(9):e022404.

220. Tzivian L, Winkler A, et al. Effect of long-term outdoor air pollution and noise on cognitive and psychological functions in adults. *Int J Hyg Environ Health.* 2015 Jan;218(1):1-11.

221. Tzivian L, Jokisch M, et al. Associations of long-term exposure to air pollution and road traffic noise with cognitive function-An analysis of effect measure modification. *Environ Int.* 2017 Jun;103:30-38.

222. Weuve J. Invited commentary: how exposure to air pollution may shape dementia risk, and what epidemiology can say about it. *Am J Epidemiol.* 2014 Aug 15;180(4):367-71.

223. See, for example:

Hyppönen E, Berry D, et al. 25-Hydroxyvitamin D and pre-clinical alterations in inflammatory and hemostatic markers: a cross sectional analysis in the 1958 British Birth Cohort. *PLoS One.* 2010 May 24;5(5):e10801.

Blondon M, Cushman M, et al. Associations of serum 25-hydroxyvitamin d with hemostatic and inflammatory biomarkers in the multi-ethnic study of atherosclerosis. *J Clin Endocrinol Metab.* 2016 Jun;101(6):2348-57.

Faridi KF, Lupton JR, et al. Vitamin D deficiency and non-lipid biomarkers of cardiovascular risk. *Arch Med Sci.* 2017 Jun;13(4):732-737.

224. Dowdy JC, Sayre RM, Holick MF. Holick's rule and vitamin D from sunlight. *J Steroid Biochem Mol Biol.* 2010 Jul; 121(1-2):328-30.

225. Holick MF. Vitamin D deficiency. *N Engl J Med. 2007* Jul 19;357(3):266-81.

226. See, for example: Meyer P, Guiraud T, et al. Exposure to extreme cold lowers the ischemic threshold in coronary artery disease patients. *Can J Cardiol.* 2010 Feb;26(2):e50-3.

227. Larra MF, Schilling TM, et al. Enhanced stress response by a bilateral feet compared to a unilateral hand Cold Pressor Test. *Stress.* 2015;18(5):589-96.

228. Sartini C, Barry SJ, et al. Relationship between outdoor temperature and cardiovascular disease risk factors in older people. *Eur J Prev Cardiol.* 2017 Mar;24(4):349-356.

229. Mitchell Dr, Derakhshan MH, et al. Abdominal compression by waist belt aggravates gastroesophageal reflux, primarily by impairing esophageal clearance. *Gastroenterology.* 2017 Jun;152(8):1881-1888.

230. Lüddecke R, Lindner T, etc. Should you stop wearing neckties?-wearing a tight necktie reduces cerebral blood flow. *Neuroradiology.* 2018 Aug;60(8):861-864.

231. See, for example: Rechner AR, Kroner C. Anthocyanins and colonic metabolites of dietary polyphenols inhibit platelet function. *Thromb Res.* 2005;116(4):327-34.

232. Consider the following examples:

   Zhu F, Du B, Xu B. Anti-inflammatory effects of phytochemicals from fruits, vegetables, and food legumes: A review. *Crit Rev Food Sci Nutr.* 2018 May 24;58(8):1260-1270.

   Watzl B. Anti-inflammatory effects of plant-based foods and of their constituents. *Int J Vitam Nutr Res.* 2008 Dec;78(6):293-8.

   Slavin JL, Lloyd B. Health benefits of fruits and vegetables. *Adv Nutr.* 2012 Jul 1;3(4):506-16.

   Alexander S, Ostfeld RJ, et al. A plant-based diet and hypertension. *J Geriatr Cardiol.* 2017 May;14(5):327-330.

   James S, Vorster HH, et al. Nutritional status influences plasma fibrinogen concentration: evidence from the THUSA survey. *Thromb Res.* 2000 Jun 1;98(5):383-94.

   Wannamethee SG, Lowe GD, et al. Associations of vitamin C status, fruit and vegetable intakes, and markers of inflammation and hemostasis. *Am J Clin Nutr.* 2006 Mar;83(3):567-74.

   Galleano M, Pechanova O, Fraga CG. Hypertension, nitric oxide, oxidants, and dietary plant polyphenols. *Curr Pharm Biotechnol.* 2010 Dec;11(8):837-48.

   Turner-McGrievy GM, Wirth MD, et al. Randomization to plant-based dietary approaches leads to larger short-term improvements in Dietary Inflammatory Index scores and macronutrient intake compared with diets that contain meat. *Nutr Res.* 2015 Feb;35(2):97-106.

   Srinivasan M, Sudheer AR, Menon VP. Ferulic Acid: therapeutic potential through its antioxidant property. *J Clin Biochem Nutr.* 2007 Mar;40(2):92-100.

233. Gorudko IV, Shamova EV, et al. Glutathione-dependent regulation of platelet aggregation with neutrophils and tumor cells [English abstract]. *Biofizika.* 2012 Jan-Feb;57(1):93-8.

234. Lampe JW. Health effects of vegetables and fruit: assessing mechanisms of action in human experimental studies. *Am J Clin Nutr*. 1999 Sep;70(3 Suppl):475S-490S.

235. Lidder S, Webb AJ. Vascular effects of dietary nitrate (as found in green leafy vegetables and beetroot) via the nitrate-nitrite-nitric oxide pathway. *Br J Clin Pharmacol*. 2013 Mar;75(3):677-96.

236. Okita M, Sasagawa T, et al. Green vegetable juice increases polyunsaturated fatty acid of erythrocyte membrane phospholipid in hypercholesterolaemic patients. *Asia Pac J Clin Nutr*. 2000 Dec;9(4):309-13.

237. United States Department of Agriculture (USDA). All about the vegetable group. https://www.choosemyplate.gov/vegetables. Updated 3 January 2018. Accessed 24 November 2018.

238. Foster-Powell K, Holt SH, Brand-Miller JC. International table of glycemic index and glycemic load values: 2002. *Am J Clin Nutr*. 2002 Jul;76(1):5-56.

239. Venn BJ, Green TJ. Glycemic index and glycemic load: measurement issues and their effect on diet-disease relationships. *Eur J Clin Nutr*. 2007 Dec;61 Suppl 1:S122-31.

240. Available free of charge at: www.compasshealth.net/diabetes-food-handout/.

241. Seringec N, Guncu G, et al. Investigation of hemorheological parameters in periodontal diseases. *Clin Hemorheol Microcirc*. 2015;61(1):47-58.

242. U.S. Centers for Disease Control and Prevention (CDC). Periodontal disease. https://www.cdc.gov/oralhealth/periodontal_disease/index.htm. Updated 10 March 2015. Accessed 24 November 2018.

243. The Cleveland Clinic. Gingivitis and periodontal disease (Gum disease). https://my.clevelandclinic.org/health/diseases/10950-gingivitis-and-periodontal-disease-gum-disease. Updated 2 May 2017. Accessed 24 November 2018.

244. U.S. Centers for Disease Control and Prevention (CDC). Periodontal disease. Op. cit.

245. American Dental Association (ADA) Division of Science. For the patient. Keeping your gums healthy. *J Am Dent Assoc*. 2015 Apr;146(4):A46.

246. The Cleveland Clinic. Gingivitis and periodontal disease (Gum disease): Prevention. https://my.clevelandclinic.org/health/diseases/10950-gingivitis-and-periodontal-disease-gum-disease/prevention. Updated 2 May 2017. Accessed 24 November 2018.

247. Pokusa M, Kráľová Trančíková A. The central role of biometals maintains oxidative balance in the context of metabolic and neurodegenerative disorders. *Oxid Med Cell Longev.* 2017;2017:8210734.

248. Dong JF, Cruz MA, et al. Magnesium maintains endothelial integrity, up-regulates proteolysis of ultra-large von Willebrand factor, and reduces platelet aggregation under flow conditions. *Thromb Haemost.* 2008 Mar;99(3):586-93.

249. Rebholz CM, Tin A, et al. Dietary magnesium and kidney function decline: The healthy aging in neighborhoods of diversity across the life span study. *Am J Nephrol.* 2016;44(5):381-387.

250. Scheibe F, Haupt H, Vlastos GA. Preventive magnesium supplement reduces ischemia-induced hearing loss and blood viscosity in the guinea pig. *Eur Arch Otorhinolaryngol.* 2000;257(7):355-61.

251. Choi YH, Miller JM, et al. Antioxidant vitamins and magnesium and the risk of hearing loss in the US general population. *Am J Clin Nutr.* 2014 Jan;99(1):148-55.

252. DeRose D, Steinke G, Li T. *Thirty Days to Natural Blood Pressure Control: The "No Pressure" Solution.* 2016. Foresthill, CA: CompassHealth Consulting Press, p. 85-6.

253. Gommers LM, Hoenderop JG, et al. Hypomagnesemia in type 2 diabetes: A vicious circle? *Diabetes.* 2016 Jan;65(1):3-13.

254. Malavade P, Hiremath S. Proton pump inhibitors: More indigestion than relief? *Indian J Nephrol.* 2017 Jul-Aug;27(4):249-257.

255. Kieboom BC, Kiefte-de Jong JC, et al. Proton pump inhibitors and hypomagnesemia in the general population: a population-based cohort study. *Am J Kidney Dis.* 2015 Nov;66(5):775-82.

256. Therapeutic Research Faculty 2018. Magnesium: Uses, side effects, interactions, dosage, and warnings. *WebMD.* https://www.webmd.com/vitamins/ai/ingredientmono-998/magnesium. Published 2018. Accessed 24 November 2018.

257. DeRose D, Steinke G, Li T. *Thirty Days to Natural Blood Pressure Control: The "No Pressure" Solution.* 2016. Foresthill, CA: CompassHealth Consulting Press, p. 251-254.

258. Kass L, Weekes J, Carpenter L. Effect of magnesium supplementation on blood pressure: a meta-analysis. *Eur J Clin Nutr.* 2012 Apr;66(4):411-8.

259. Office of Dietary Supplements (U.S. Department of Health & Human Services). Magnesium: Fact sheet for health professionals. https://ods.od.nih.gov/factsheets/Magnesium-HealthProfessional/#h7. Updated 26 September 2018. Accessed 24 November 2018.

260. See, for example:

Jiang W, Boyle SH, et al. Platelet aggregation and mental stress induced myocardial ischemia: Results from the Responses of Myocardial Ischemia to Escitalopram Treatment (REMIT) study. *Am Heart J.* 2015 Apr;169(4):496-507.

Bairey Merz CN, Dwyer J, et al. Psychosocial stress and cardiovascular disease: pathophysiological links. *Behav Med.* 2002 Winter;27(4):141-7.

Wenneberg SR, Schneider RH, et al. Anger expression correlates with platelet aggregation. *Behav Med.* 1997 Winter;22(4):174-7.

261. Romans 1:14. *The Holy Bible: English Standard Version.* 2001. Wheaton, IL: Standard Bible Society.

262. Philippians 2:3. *The Holy Bible: English Standard Version.* 2001. Wheaton, IL: Standard Bible Society.

263. Coulehan J. On humility. *Ann Intern Med.* 2010 Aug 3;153(3):200-1.

264. Stein T. Humility: The art of self-forgetfulness. http://blogs.bible.org/engage/tiffany_stein/humility_the_art_of_self-forgetfulness. Published 18 March 2015. Accessed 24 November 2018.

265. Howard R, Lash J. *This Was Your Life! Preparing to Meet God Face to Face.* 1998. Grand Rapids, MI: Chosen Books, p. 85.

266. See, for example:

Lewis TT, Aiello AE, et al. Self-reported experiences of everyday discrimination are associated with elevated C-reactive protein levels in older African-American adults. *Brain Behav Immun.* 2010;24(3):438–443.

Kershaw KN, Lewis TT, et al. Self-reported experiences of discrimination and inflammation among men and women: The multi-ethnic study of atherosclerosis. *Health Psychol.* 2016 Apr;35(4):343-50.

267. See, for example:

Redwine LS, Henry BL, et al. Pilot randomized study of a gratitude journaling intervention on heart rate variability and inflammatory biomarkers in patients with Stage B heart failure. *Psychosom Med.* 2016 Jul-Aug;78(6):667-76.

Moieni M, Irwin MR, et al. Exploring the role of gratitude and support-giving on inflammatory outcomes. *Emotion.* 2018 Sep 27. doi: 10.1037/emo0000472. [Epub ahead of print].

268. See, for example:

Sirois FM, Wood AM. Gratitude uniquely predicts lower depression in chronic illness populations: A longitudinal study of inflammatory bowel disease and arthritis. *Health Psychol.* 2017 Feb;36(2):122-132.

Henning M, Fox GR, et al. A potential role for mu-opioids in mediating the positive effects of gratitude. *Front Psychol.* 2017 Jun 21;8:868.

Anisman H, Merali Z. Cytokines, stress and depressive illness: brain-immune interactions. *Ann Med.* 2003;35(1):2-11.

269. Aksungar FB, Topkaya AE, Akyildiz M. Interleukin-6, C-reactive protein and biochemical parameters during prolonged intermittent fasting. *Ann Nutr Metab.* 2007;51(1):88-95.

270. Faris MA, Kacimi S, et al. Intermittent fasting during Ramadan attenuates proinflammatory cytokines and immune cells in healthy subjects. *Nutr Res.* 2012 Dec;32(12):947-55.

271. Unalacak M, Kara IH, et al. Effects of Ramadan fasting on biochemical and hematological parameters and cytokines in healthy and obese individuals. *Metab Syndr Relat Disord.* 2011 Apr;9(2):157-61.

272. Moro T, Tinsley G, et al. Effects of eight weeks of time-restricted feeding (16/8) on basal metabolism, maximal strength, body composition, inflammation, and cardiovascular risk factors in resistance-trained males. *J Transl Med.* 2016;14(1):290.

273. DeRose DJ, Charles-Marcel ZL, et al. Vegan-based lifestyle for diabetic neuropathy: A model for managed care. Presented at the American Public Health Association's 126th Annual Meeting; Washington, D.C. November 1998.

274. See, for example:

Williams KV, Mullen ML, et al. The effect of short periods of caloric restriction on weight loss and glycemic control in type 2 diabetes. *Diabetes Care*. 1998 Jan;21(1):2-8.

Goldhamer A, Lisle D, et al. Medically supervised water-only fasting in the treatment of hypertension. *J Manipulative Physiol Ther*. 2001 Jun;24(5):335-9.

275. See, for example:

Salomaa V, Rasi V, et al. The effects of saturated fat and n-6 polyunsaturated fat on postprandial lipemia and hemostatic activity. *Atherosclerosis*. 1993 Oct;103(1):1-11.

Tholstrup T, Miller GJ, et al. Effect of individual dietary fatty acids on postprandial activation of blood coagulation factor VII and fibrinolysis in healthy young men. *Am J Clin Nutr*. 2003 May;77(5):1125-32.

276. Cunningham W, Hyson D. The skinny on high-protein, low-carbohydrate diets. *Prev Cardiol*. 2006 Summer;9(3):166-71.

277. Russell WR, Gratz SW, et al. High-protein, reduced-carbohydrate weight-loss diets promote metabolite profiles likely to be detrimental to colonic health. *Am J Clin Nutr*. 2011 May;93(5):1062-72.

278. Chiba M, Tsuda S, et al. Onset of ulcerative colitis during a low-carbohydrate weight-loss diet and treatment with a plant-based diet: A case report. *Perm J*. 2016 Winter;20(1):80-4.

279. Wong A. Pandemonium and rage in Hawaii. *The Atlantic*. https://www.theatlantic.com/international/archive/2018/01/pandemonium-and-rage-in-hawaii/550529/. 14 January 2018. Accessed on 25 November 2018.

280. For an example of perceived stress in the face of financial stressors, see: Whitehead BR, Bergeman CS. The effect of the financial crisis on physical health: Perceived impact matters. *J Health Psychol*. 2017 Jun;22(7):864-873.

281. Koudouovoh-Tripp P, Sperner-Unterweger B. Influence of mental stress on platelet bioactivity. *World J Psychiatry*. 2012 Dec 22;2(6):134-47.

282. Wei Jiang, Stephen H. Boyle, et al. Platelet aggregation and mental stress induced myocardial ischemia: Results from the REMIT study. *Am Heart J*. 2015 Apr; 169(4): 496–507.

283. See, for example: Strawbridge WJ, Shema SJ, et al. Religious attendance increases survival by improving and maintaining good health behaviors, mental health, and social relationships. *Ann Behav Med.* 2001 Winter;23(1):68-74.

284. The *Changing Bad Habits for Good* DVD is available at www.compass-health.net/purchase.

285. *30 Days to Natural Diabetes and High Blood Pressure Control* is easy to access from the Free Materials section on the CompassHealth.net website: www.compasshealth.net/diabetes-bp/. Alternately you can access it directly on YouTube under *NEW, REVISED – 30 Days to Natural Diabetes and High Blood Pressure Control* at https://www.youtube.com/playlist?list=PLW2SvLyeNKrSgx8l6TiBefPPaCw8j-j1i.

286. Ephesians 4:26. *The Holy Bible: King James Version* (electronic ed. of the 1769 edition of the 1611 Authorized Version). Bellingham, WA: Logos Research Systems, Inc.

287. You can access archived broadcasts at: https://www.americanindianliving.org/.

288. Cheong EV, Sinnott C, et al. Adverse childhood experiences (ACEs) and later-life depression: perceived social support as a potential protective factor. *BMJ Open.* 2017;7(9):e013228.

289. Felitti VJ, Anda RF, et al. Relationship of childhood abuse and household dysfunction to many of the leading causes of death in adults. The Adverse Childhood Experiences (ACE) Study. *Am J Prev Med.* 1998 May;14(4):245-58.

290. See, for example:

Jakubowski KP, Cundiff JM, Matthews KA. Cumulative childhood adversity and adult cardiometabolic disease: A meta-analysis. *Health Psychol.* 2018 Aug;37(8):701-715.

Hughes K, Bellis MA, et al. The effect of multiple adverse childhood experiences on health: a systematic review and meta-analysis. *Lancet Public Health.* 2017 Aug;2(8):e356-e366.

Gilbert LK, Breiding MJ, et al. Childhood adversity and adult chronic disease: an update from ten states and the District of Columbia, 2010. *Am J Prev Med.* 2015 Mar;48(3):345-9.

Felitti VJ, Anda RF, et al. Op. cit.

291. Kalmakis KA, Meyer JS, et al. Adverse childhood experiences and chronic hypothalamic-pituitary-adrenal activity. *Stress*. 2015;18(4):446-50.

292. Zhu LJ, Liu MY, et al. The different roles of glucocorticoids in the hippocampus and hypothalamus in chronic stress-induced HPA axis hyperactivity. *PLoS One*. 2014 May 15;9(5):e97689.

293. For example, see:

Sirois FM, Hirsch JK. A longitudinal study of the profiles of psychological thriving, resilience, and loss in people with inflammatory bowel disease. *Br J Health Psychol*. 2017 Nov;22(4):920-939.

Shand LK, Cowlishaw S, et al. Correlates of post-traumatic stress symptoms and growth in cancer patients: a systematic review and meta-analysis. *Psychooncology*. 2015 Jun;24(6):624-34.

Rzeszutek M, Oniszczenko W, Firląg-Burkacka E. Social support, stress coping strategies, resilience and posttraumatic growth in a Polish sample of HIV-infected individuals: results of a 1 year longitudinal study. *J Behav Med*. 2017 Dec;40(6):942-954.

Sirois FM, Hirsch JK. Associations of psychological thriving with coping efficacy, expectations for future growth, and depressive symptoms over time in people with arthritis. *J Psychosom Res*. 2013 Sep;75(3):279-86.

294. Kraft TL, Pressman SD. Grin and bear it: The influence of manipulated facial expression on the stress response. *Psychol Sci*. 2012;23(11):1372-8.

295. Lewis MB. The interactions between botulinum-toxin-based facial treatments and embodied emotions. *Sci Rep*. 2018 Oct 3;8(1):14720.

296. Epton T, Harris PR, et al. The impact of self-affirmation on health-behavior change: a meta-analysis. *Health Psychol*. 2015 Mar;34(3):187-96.

297. Ogedegbe GO, Boutin-Foster C, et al. A randomized controlled trial of positive-affect intervention and medication adherence in hypertensive African Americans. *Arch Intern Med*. 2012 Feb 27;172(4):322-6.

298. Armitage CJ, Harris PR, et al. Self-affirmation increases acceptance of health-risk information among UK adult smokers with low socioeconomic status. *Psychol Addict Behav*. 2008 Mar;22(1):88-95.

299. Smith R. Tributes flow for Sam Ballard, who died after eating a slug. *The New Zealand Herald*. https://www.nzherald.co.nz/world/news/article.cfm?c_id=2&objectid=12155407. 6 Nov 2018. Accessed 25 November 2018.

300. For more information about this microbe, see: Murphy GS, Johnson S. Clinical aspects of eosinophilic meningitis and meningoencephalitis caused by Angiostrongylus cantonensis, the rat lungworm. *Hawaii J Med Public Health*. 2013 Jun;72(6 Suppl 2):35-40.

301. Conlon MJ. FDA warns against herbal remedies. *UPI Archives*. https://www.upi.com/Archives/1980/12/15/FDA-warns-against-herbal-remedies/1924345704400/. 15 December 1980. Accessed 25 November 2018.

302. See, for example: Breeher L, Mikulski MA, et al. A cluster of lead poisoning among consumers of Ayurvedic medicine. *Int J Occup Environ Health*. 2015;21(4):303-7.

303. Examples include:

Kasperczyk A, Słowińska-Łożyńska L, et al. The effect of lead-induced oxidative stress on blood viscosity and rheological properties of erythrocytes in lead exposed humans. *Clin Hemorheol Microcirc*. 2014;56(3):187–95.

Chowdhury R, Ramond A, et al. Environmental toxic metal contaminants and risk of cardiovascular disease: systematic review and meta-analysis. *BMJ*. 2018 Aug 29;362:k3310.

Jomova K, Valko M. Advances in metal-induced oxidative stress and human disease. *Toxicology*. 2011 May 10;283(2-3):65-87.

Alissa EM, Ferns GA. Heavy metal poisoning and cardiovascular disease. *J Toxicol*. 2011;2011:870125.

304. Clénin GE. The treatment of iron deficiency without anaemia (in otherwise healthy persons). *Swiss Med Wkly*. 2017 Jun 14;147:w14434.

305. See, for example:

Mannaerts D, Faes E, et al. Oxidative stress in healthy pregnancy and preeclampsia is linked to chronic inflammation, iron status and vascular function. *PLoS One*. 2018 Sep 11;13(9):e0202919.

Gutierrez-Aguirre CH, García-Lozano JA, et al. Comparative analysis of iron status and other hematological parameters in preeclampsia. *Hematology*. 2017 Jan;22(1):36-40.

Kataria Y, Wu Y, et al. Iron status and gestational diabetes-a meta-analysis. *Nutrients*. 2018 May 15;10(5).

Kim J, Kim YJ, et al. Serum levels of zinc, calcium, and iron are associated with the risk of preeclampsia in pregnant women. *Nutr Res.* 2012 Oct;32(10):764-9.

Siddiqui IA, Jaleel A, et al. Iron status parameters in preeclamptic women. *Arch Gynecol Obstet.* 2011 Sep;284(3):587-91.

306. Cohen PA, Wen A, Gerona R. Prohibited Stimulants in dietary supplements after enforcement action by the US Food and Drug Administration. *JAMA Intern Med.* Published online 22 October 2018. doi: 10.1001/jamainternmed.2018.4846. [Epub ahead of print].

307. Cohen PA, Travis JC, et al. The stimulant higenamine in weight loss and sports supplements. *Clin Toxicol (Phila).* 2018 Sep 6:1-6.

308. Mayo Clinic Staff. Medications and supplements that can raise your blood pressure. *Mayo Clinic On-line.* http://www.mayoclinic.org/diseases-conditions/high-blood-pressure/in-depth/blood-pressure/art-20045245?pg=2. Updated 11 February 2016. Accessed 25 November 2018.

309. Cohen PA, Wen A, Gerona R. Op. Cit.

310. Ekabe CJ, Kehbila J, et al. Vitamin B12 deficiency neuropathy; a rare diagnosis in young adults: a case report. *BMC Res Notes.* 2017 Jan 28;10(1):72.

311. U.S. Centers for Disease Control and Prevention (CDC). Vitamin B12 deficiency in resettled Bhutanese refugees--United States, 2008-2011. *MMWR Morb Mortal Wkly Rep.* 2011 Mar 25;60(11):343-6.

312. Allen LH. How common is vitamin B-12 deficiency? *Am J Clin Nutr.* 2009 Feb;89(2):693S-6S.

313. Tancer-Elci H, Isik-Balci Y, et al. Investigation of hemorheological parameters at the diagnosis and the follow-up of nutritional vitamin B12 deficient children. *Clin Hemorheol Microcirc.* 2015;60(3):273-82.

314. See, for example: Rizzo G, Laganà AS, et al. Vitamin B12 among vegetarians: Status, assessment and supplementation. *Nutrients.* 2016;8(12):767.

315. Office of Dietary Supplements (U.S. Department of Health & Human Services). Omega-3 fatty acids and health: Fact sheet for health professionals. https://ods.od.nih.gov/factsheets/Omega3FattyAcidsandHealth-HealthProfessional/ . Updated 28 October 2005. Accessed 25 November 2018.

316. McEwen BJ, Morel-Kopp MC, et al. Effects of omega-3 polyunsaturated fatty acids on platelet function in healthy subjects and subjects with cardiovascular disease. *Semin Thromb Hemost*. 2013 Feb;39(1):25-32.

317. Menon S. Mercury guide. *Natural Resources Defense Council*. https://www.nrdc.org/stories/mercury-guide. 10 March 2016. Accessed 25 November 2018.

318. Hu XF, Laird BD, Chan HM. Mercury diminishes the cardiovascular protective effect of omega-3 polyunsaturated fatty acids in the modern diet of Inuit in Canada. *Environ Res*. 2017 Jan;152:470-477.

319. Connor WE, Connor, SL. Omega-3 fatty acids from fish (Chapter 12). In Bendich A, Deckelbaum RJ, eds. *Preventive Nutrition: The Comprehensive Guide for Health Professionals*. 1997. New York: Humana Press, p. 225-243.

320. DeRose D, Steinke G, Li T. *Thirty Days to Natural Blood Pressure Control: The "No Pressure" Solution*. 2016. Foresthill, CA: CompassHealth Consulting Press, p. 260-263.

321. Bonaventura P, Benedetti G, et al. Zinc and its role in immunity and inflammation. *Autoimmun Rev*. 2015 Apr;14(4):277-85.

322. Pokusa M, Kráľová Trančíková A. The Central Role of Biometals Maintains Oxidative Balance in the Context of Metabolic and Neurodegenerative Disorders. *Oxid Med Cell Longev*. 2017;2017:8210734.

323. See, for example: Kim J, Kim YJ, et al. Serum levels of zinc, calcium, and iron are associated with the risk of preeclampsia in pregnant women. *Nutr Res*. 2012 Oct;32(10):764-9.

324. See, for example: Islam MA, Alam F, et al. Natural products towards the discovery of potential future antithrombotic drugs. *Curr Pharm Des*. 2016;22(20):2926-46.

325. Examples include:

    Li AN, Li S, et al. Resources and biological activities of natural polyphenols. *Nutrients*. 2014 Dec 22;6(12):6020-47.

    Islam MA, Alam F, et al. Dietary phytochemicals: Natural swords combating inflammation and oxidation-mediated degenerative diseases. *Oxid Med Cell Longev*. 2016;2016:5137431.

326. Blodgett B. *A Message from Jessie: The Incredible True Story of Murder and Miracles in the Heartland*. 2015. Los Angeles, CA: Story Merchant Books.

327. Jones LG. Living forgiveness: Lessons on the fifth anniversary of the Amish schoolhouse shootings. *The Baltimore Sun*. https://www.baltimoresun.com/news/opinion/oped/bs-ed-amish-forgiveness-20111002-story.html. Published 2 October 2011. Accessed 25 November 2018.

328. See, for example: ten Boom C. Guideposts classics: Corrie ten Boom on forgiveness. *Guideposts*. https://www.guideposts.org/better-living/positive-living/guideposts-classics-corrie-ten-boom-on-forgiveness. Posted 24 July 2014. Accessed 25 November 2018.

329. Stableford D. Families of Charleston shooting victims to Dylann Roof: We forgive you. *Yahoo News*. https://news.yahoo.com/familes-of-charleston-church-shooting-victims-to-dylann-roof--we--forgive-you-185833509.html. Published 19 June 2015. Accessed 25 November 2018.

330. DeRose D, Blodget B. A Message from Jessie. *American Indian Living Radio*. https://soundcloud.com/americanindianliving/buck-blodgett-podcast. Published 30 January 2017. Accessed 25 November 2018.

331. Martin B. Getting anger and hostility under control. *Psych Central*. https://psychcentral.com/lib/getting-anger-and-hostility-under-control/. Updated 17 July 2016. Accessed 25 November 2018.

332. See, for example:

Jiang W, Boyle SH, et al. Platelet aggregation and mental stress induced myocardial ischemia: Results from the Responses of Myocardial Ischemia to Escitalopram Treatment (REMIT) study. *Am Heart J*. 2015 Apr;169(4):496-507.

Bairey Merz CN, Dwyer J, et al. Psychosocial stress and cardiovascular disease: pathophysiological links. *Behav Med*. 2002 Winter;27(4):141-7.

Wenneberg SR, Schneider RH, et al. Anger expression correlates with platelet aggregation. *Behav Med*. 1997 Winter;22(4):174-7.

333. Von Känel R, Vökt F, et al. Relation of psychological distress to the international normalized ratio in patients with venous thromboembolism with and without oral anticoagulant therapy. *J Thromb Haemost*. 2012 Aug;10(8):1547-55.

334. Irish AB, Green FR. Factor VII coagulant activity (VIIc) and hypercoagulability in chronic renal disease and dialysis: relationship with dyslipidaemia, inflammation, and factor VII genotype. *Nephrol Dial Transplant*. 1998 Mar;13(3):679-84.

335. Boylan JM, Lewis TT, et al. Educational status, anger, and inflammation in the MIDUS national sample: Does race matter? *Ann Behav Med.* 2015 Aug;49(4):570-8.

336. Ranjit N, Diez-Roux AV, et al. Psychosocial factors and inflammation in the multi-ethnic study of atherosclerosis. *Arch Intern Med.* 2007 Jan 22;167(2):174-81.

337. Goldstein S, Goldstein E. Let it go: 11 ways to forgive. *Mindful (Magazine).* https://www.mindful.org/let-go-11-ways-forgive/. Published 20 March 2017. Accessed 25 November 2018.

338. Valeo T. Forgive and forget. *WebMD Archives.* https://www.webmd.com/mental-health/features/forgive-forget#1. Published 9 February 2007. Accessed 25 November 2018.

339. DeRose D, Steinke G, Li T. *Thirty Days to Natural Blood Pressure Control: The "No Pressure" Solution.* 2016. Foresthill, CA: CompassHealth Consulting Press, p. 339.

340. The Greater Good Science Center at UC Berkeley. What is forgiveness? *Greater Good Magazine.* https://greatergood.berkeley.edu/topic/forgiveness/definition. Accessed 25 November 2018.

341. Rowland L, Curry OS. A range of kindness activities boost happiness. *J Soc Psychol.* 2018 Apr 27:1-4.

342. See, for example:

DuBois CM, Millstein RA, et al. Feasibility and acceptability of a positive psychological intervention for patients with type 2 diabetes. *Prim Care Companion CNS Disord.* 2016;18(3):10.4088/PCC.15m01902.

Boehm JK, Soo J, et al. Longitudinal associations between psychological well-being and the consumption of fruits and vegetables. *Health Psychol.* 2018 Oct;37(10):959-967.

343. See, for example: von Känel R, Kudielka BM, et al. Opposite effect of negative and positive affect on stress procoagulant reactivity. *Physiol Behav.* 2005 Sep 15;86(1-2):61-8.

344. Random Acts of Kindness. Kindness ideas. https://www.randomactsofkindness.org/kindness-ideas. Accessed 25 November 2018.

345. Random Acts. Kindness ideas: No matter how much time you have, there's always time to be kind. https://www.randomacts.org/kindness-ideas/. Accessed 25 November 2018.

346. Xie Z, Chen F, et al. A review of sleep disorders and melatonin. *Neurol Res.* 2017 Jun;39(6):559-565.

347. Baltatu OC, Amaral FG, et al. Melatonin, mitochondria and hypertension. *Cell Mol Life Sci.* 2017 Nov;74(21):3955-3964.

348. Grossman E, Laudon M, Zisapel N. Effect of melatonin on nocturnal blood pressure: meta-analysis of randomized controlled trials. *Vasc Health Risk Manag.* 2011;7:577-84.

349. Bonomini F, Borsani E, et al. Dietary melatonin supplementation could be a promising preventing/therapeutic approach for a variety of liver diseases. *Nutrients.* 2018 Aug 21;10(9):1135.

350. See, for example:

Mozaffari S, Rahimi R, Abdollahi M. Implications of melatonin therapy in irritable bowel syndrome: a systematic review. *Curr Pharm Des.* 2010;16(33):3646-55.

Chen CQ, Fichna J, et al. Distribution, function and physiological role of melatonin in the lower gut. *World J Gastroenterol.* 2011 Sep 14;17(34):3888-98.

351. Li Y, Li S, et al. Melatonin for the prevention and treatment of cancer. *Oncotarget.* 2017 Jun 13;8(24):39896-39921.

352. Bondy SC, Campbell A. Mechanisms underlying tumor suppressive properties of melatonin. *Int J Mol Sci.* 2018 Jul 27;19(8):2205.

353. Carrillo-Vico A, Guerrero JM, et al. A review of the multiple actions of melatonin on the immune system. *Endocrine.* 2005 Jul;27(2):189-200.

354. Bonnefont-Rousselot D, Collin F. Melatonin: action as antioxidant and potential applications in human disease and aging. *Toxicology.* 2010 Nov 28;278(1):55-67.

355. Gagnon K, Godbout R. Melatonin and comorbidities in children with autism spectrum disorder. *Curr Dev Disord Rep.* 2018;5(3):197-206.

356. Masters A, Pandi-Perumal SR, et al. Melatonin, the hormone of darkness: From sleep promotion to Ebola treatment. *Brain Disord Ther.* 2014;4(1):1000151.

357. Wirtz PH, Spillmann M, et al. Oral melatonin reduces blood coagulation activity: a placebo-controlled study in healthy young men. *J Pineal Res.* 2008 Mar;44(2):127-33.

358. Wirtz PH, Bärtschi C, et al. Effect of oral melatonin on the procoagulant response to acute psychosocial stress in healthy men: a randomized placebo-controlled study. *J Pineal Res*. 2008 May;44(4):358-65.

359. Zhang L, Gong JT, et al. melatonin attenuates noise stress-induced gastrointestinal motility disorder and gastric stress ulcer: Role of gastrointestinal hormones and oxidative stress in rats. *J Neurogastroenterol Motil*. 2015 Mar 30;21(2):189-99.

360. Sirtori CR, Arnoldi A, Cicero AF. Nutraceuticals for blood pressure control. *Ann Med*. 2015 Sep 11:1-10.

361. Grossman E, Laudon M, Zisapel N. Effect of melatonin on nocturnal blood pressure: meta-analysis of randomized controlled trials. *Vasc Health Risk Manag*. 2011;7:577-84.

362. Wurtman R. Physiology and available preparations of melatonin. *UpToDate*. Updated 17 April 2017. Accessed 18 November 2018.

363. Zhdanova IV, Wurtman RJ, et al. Effects of low oral doses of melatonin, given 2-4 hours before habitual bedtime, on sleep in normal young humans. *Sleep*. 1996 Jun;19(5):423-31.

364. Lyseng-Williamson KA. Melatonin prolonged release: in the treatment of insomnia in patients aged ≥55 years. *Drugs Aging*. 2012 Nov;29(11):911-23.

365. Bertrand PP, Polglaze KE, et al. Detection of melatonin production from the intestinal epithelium using electrochemical methods. *Curr Pharm Des*. 2014;20(30):4802-6.

366. Thor PJ, Krolczyk G, et al. Melatonin and serotonin effects on gastrointestinal motility. *J Physiol Pharmacol*. 2007 Dec;58 Suppl 6:97-103.

367. Arnao MB, Hernández-Ruiz J. The potential of phytomelatonin as a nutraceutical. *Molecules*. 2018 Jan 22;23(1):238.

368. Masters A, Pandi-Perumal SR, et al. Melatonin, the hormone of darkness: From sleep promotion to Ebola treatment. *Brain Disord Ther*. 2014;4(1):1000151.

369. Nedley N. Melatonin: Agent for rest and rejuvenation (Chapter 9). In *Proof Positive: How to Reliably Combat Disease and Achieve Optimal Health Through Nutrition and Lifestyle*. 1998. Ardmore, OK: Nedley Publishing, p. 193-210.

370. For example, see:

Wurtman R. Physiology and available preparations of melatonin. *UpToDate*. Updated 17 April 2017. Accessed 18 November 2018.

Arnao MB, Hernández-Ruiz J. The potential of phytomelatonin as a nutraceutical. *Molecules*. 2018 Jan 22;23(1):238.

371. For example, see:

Ornish D, Brown SE, et al. Can lifestyle changes reverse coronary heart disease? The Lifestyle Heart Trial. *Lancet*. 1990 Jul 21;336(8708):129-33.

Ornish D, Scherwitz LW, et al. Intensive lifestyle changes for reversal of coronary heart disease. *JAMA*. 1998 Dec 16;280(23):2001-7.

372. Full details on how to run an eight-session high blood pressure seminar are found at: www.compasshealth.net/hypertension/. The program can be run twice per week for four weeks, or once weekly for eight weeks. It uses our book, *Thirty Days to Natural Blood Pressure Control*, along with four DVDs: *Changing Bad Habits for Good*, *Reversing Hypertension Naturally*, *Listening to the Buffalo*, and *Spiritual Health: Neglected Dimensions*.

INDEX

Numbers

A

B

Bad-habit glue 120
Bad habits 94, 229, 314, 323
Baldwin, Bernell v, 120, 122
Bean(s) 110, 111, 115, 140
Bedroom location 143, 184, 240, 244, 259
Behaviors 89, 161, 213, 229, 233, 239, 266, 314
Blindness 31, 33, 60
Blodgett, Buck 259, 260, 318
Blood bank 51, 86, 87, 93, 96, 97, 98, 212, 257
Blood donation 50, 51, 96, 97, 98, 139, 140, 212, 257, 269, 292, 297, 301
Blood donor(s) 51, 97
Blood doping 17, 77, 290
Bloodletting 212
Blood pressure xiii, 47, 50, 95, 101, 102, 113, 116, 128, 142, 154, 174, 203, 239, 249, 256, 279, 281, 285, 286, 299, 302, 303, 306, 310, 314, 318, 320, 323
Blood sugar x, 55, 87, 99, 100, 101, 102, 109, 137, 138, 144, 196, 218, 219, 273
Botox 242
Breslow, Lester 215, 216
Brushing (teeth) 201
Buteyko, Konstantin 169

C

Caerphilly 25, 41, 42, 44, 290, 292, 295
Caffeine xiv, 117, 144, 297
Caloric restriction 217, 313
Cancer 10, 35, 36, 37, 38, 39, 40, 41, 46, 94, 101, 110, 111, 119, 121, 147, 149, 238, 241, 272, 291, 298, 302, 315, 321
Changing Bad Habits for Good DVD 229, 314
Chemotherapy 241
Chia 139, 255, 256
Chiropractic 259
Choice Reaction Time (CRT) 42
Cholesterol 27, 70, 103, 184, 302
Chronic pain 154
Cigarette smoking (see also Smoking, Tobacco) 70, 171, 173, 185, 232, 238, 305
Circaseptan 125, 159, 299
Clean break(s) 122, 163, 164, 165, 180, 207
Clothing 187, 188
Cognitive performance 42, 45
Cold pressor test 188
Cold temperature(s) 188

Collagen vascular diseases 68
CompassHealth ii, 13, 86, 100, 114, 116, 142, 284, 285, 286, 309, 314, 323
Consequences 56, 74, 138, 141, 157, 232, 233, 235, 247, 297, 305
Contrast (water) treatments (see also Hydrotherapy) 155
Cooking beans 111
Cooper Institute 166
Cortisol 184, 188
Coulehan, Jack 210, 311
C-reactive protein 128, 142, 216, 261, 311, 312

D

Decisional forgiveness 265
Deep breathing 169, 170, 173, 174
Degenerative disc disease (DDD) 68
Dementia (see also Alzheimer's) ix, 45, 139, 172, 185, 305, 307
Dentist xiv, 199
Depression 184, 211, 238, 240, 241, 242, 243, 312, 314
Diabetes ix, x, 10, 31, 53, 54, 55, 56, 58, 59, 60, 61, 68, 73, 87, 96, 99, 100, 101, 102, 110, 112, 116, 129, 137, 142, 155, 171, 196, 202, 204, 218, 229, 249, 254, 284, 285, 286, 292, 293, 294, 297, 299, 304, 309, 310, 313, 314, 316, 320
Dimethylamylamine 249, 250
Dimethylbutylamine 249, 250
Distressor(s) 224, 231
DVDs 116, 279, 283, 323

E

Ear plugs 184, 188
Electrolyte(s) 150, 196
Emotional forgiveness 264, 265
Endogenous Thrombin Potential (ETP) 138, 139
Endothelium 47, 49, 173
Environment(al) 40, 144, 150, 173, 181, 182, 183, 184, 185, 186, 187, 210, 228, 232, 234
Eosinophilia-Myalgia Syndrome (EMS) 274
Ephedra 250
EPO (erythropoietin) 18, 290
Erythrocyte(s) (see also RBCs) 12, 22, 23, 200, 290, 291, 297, 306, 309, 316
Eustressor(s) 223, 224

F

Factor VII 29, 219, 261, 319

M

Macular degeneration 32, 33, 34, 35, 291
Magnesium 196, 199, 201, 202, 203, 204, 205, 206, 250, 310, 311
Ma Huang 250
Mandela, Nelson 210
Marijuana 172, 173, 174, 305
Meat(s) 121, 138, 139, 140, 197, 220, 308
Melatonin xv, 143, 144, 271, 272, 273, 274, 290, 321, 322, 323
Mercy 260
Metastasis 36, 37, 40
Minnesota 32, 95, 105, 254
Minnesota Twins 32
Mortality 37, 121, 124, 216, 290, 295, 298, 299
Motivation 6, 11, 173, 209, 232
Myocardial infarctions (MIs, see also Heart attacks) 27, 28, 290, 298, 301

N

National Wellness Conference 215
Native Americans 156, 209, 238
Natural Killer (NK) Cells 40
Nedley, Neil 274, 322
Neuropathy 155, 312, 317
NEWSTART x, 289
Nitrate(s) 194
Nitric oxide 47, 48, 49, 156, 308, 309
Noise 144, 181, 182, 183, 184, 185, 188, 306, 307, 322
Non-steroidal anti-inflammatory drugs (NSAIDs) 153
Nutrition Facts 178

O

Obesity (see also Overweight) ix, 63, 70, 111, 176, 292, 293, 294, 304
Omega-3 fat(s) 137, 139, 255, 256, 258, 317, 318
Optimism 240, 242
Osteoarthritis (OA) 70
Osteoporosis 71, 148, 206, 295
Overweight (see also Obesity) 63, 71, 86, 163, 164, 165, 166, 202
Oxidative stress 49, 57, 58, 133, 202, 257, 293, 295, 296, 316, 322

P

Pavlov 120
Peak E 273

Periodontitis (see also Gingivitis) 200, 201
Personal rights 209, 210
Physical activity 105, 106, 108, 121, 185, 297
Phytic acid 110
Phytochemical(s) 192, 193, 194
Phytoplankton 139, 256
Plasma 19, 20, 25, 29, 33, 34, 36, 44, 200, 291, 294, 295, 301, 303, 308
Platelet(s) 19, 39, 40, 49, 53, 60, 75, 111, 118, 171, 184, 194, 198, 203, 224, 225, 255, 291, 292, 293, 294, 295, 297, 305, 308, 309, 310, 311, 313, 318, 319
Pollution 184, 306
Polyunsaturated fat(s) 137, 138, 139, 255, 313
Ponce de Leon ix
Positive Psychology 239, 244
Posttraumatic growth 240, 241, 315
Potassium 129, 196, 197
Preeclampsia 139, 249, 301, 316, 317, 318
Pregnancy 139, 249, 257, 301, 316
Protein(s) 22, 23, 38, 54, 65, 128, 138, 142, 148, 216, 220, 261, 272, 301, 303, 311, 312, 313
Proton Pump Inhibitor(s) (*prazoles*) 204, 254
Puckett, Kirby 32, 33, 291

Q

Quercetin 194

R

Ramadan 217, 312
Rat lungworm 246, 316
RBCs (red blood cells, red cells) 16, 17, 19, 20, 21, 22, 23, 29, 33, 34, 36, 37, 41, 43, 44, 49, 139, 140, 146, 165, 171, 184, 195, 200, 254, 290, 292, 303, 304, 305, 306
Red cell stiffness 171, 184
Resistance exercise(s) 131, 132, 133, 134, 135, 213
Resveratrol 194
Road rage 227
Rotating shift work 126
Rugby 78, 246, 296

S

Sabbath (see Lord's Day) 124, 125, 298
Salt (see also Sodium) 95, 127, 128, 129, 299, 300
Saturated fat(s) 137, 138, 139, 313

Made in the USA
Coppell, TX
15 January 2023

11131055R10204